£29.99

77

Medicines Management in Mental Health Care

Dedications

To Toni, Myla, Zac and Hattie, who give me so much love and happiness.

To Anke, Jack, Rob and Anna.

Medicines Management in Mental Health Care

Edited by

Neil Harris, John Baker and Richard Gray

WILEY-BLACKWELL

A John Wiley & Sons, Ltd., Publication

This edition first published 2009
© 2009 Blackwell Publishing Ltd.

Wiley-Blackwell is an imprint of John Wiley & Sons, formed by the merger of Wiley's
global Scientific, Technical and Medical business with Blackwell Publishing.

Registered office
John Wiley & Sons Ltd, The Atrium, Southern Gate, Chichester, West Sussex,
PO19 8SQ, United Kingdom

Editorial office
9600 Garsington Road, Oxford, Oxt ZDQ, United Kingdom2121 State Avenue,
Arres, Iown, 50014 8300, USA

For details of our global editorial offices, for customer services and for information
about how to apply for permission to reuse the copyright material in this book please
see our website at www.wiley.com/wiley-blackwell.

Library of Congress Cataloging-in-Publication Data
Medicines management in mental health care / edited by Neil Harris, John Baker,
and Richard Gray.
p. ; cm.
Includes bibliographical references and index.
ISBN 978-1-4051-3289-3 (pbk. : alk. paper)
1. Psychotropic drugs–Administration. 2. Drugs–Prescribing. 3. Psychiatric
nursing. I. Harris, Neil, 1954- II. Baker, John, 1974- III. Gray, Richard, Dr.
[DNLM: 1. Mental Disorders–drug therapy–Great Britain. 2. Drug
Prescriptions–nursing–Great Britain. 3. Medication Therapy Management–Great
Britain. 4. Mental Disorders–nursing–Great Britain. 5. Psychotropic Drugs–
therapeutic use–Great Britain. WM 402 M489 2009]
RC483.M43 2009
362.196′86–dc22
2009005451

A catalogue record for this book is available from the British Library.

Set in 10 on 12.5 pt Palatino by SNP Best-set Typesetter Ltd., Hong Kong
Printed in Singapore by Ho Printing Singapore Pte Ltd
1   2009

Contents

The Editors

Dr Neil Harris, BSc (Hons), RNM, RGN

Since qualifying as a mental health nurse in the 1970s Neil has maintained a clinical focus to his work. He completed the Thorn PSI Diploma in 1994 and became an honorary lecturer with the University of Manchester in 1996. He was awarded a PhD from the University of Manchester in 2002. He is currently a Consultant Nurse at Manchester Mental Health and Social Care Trust and Lecturer at the University of Manchester. He has presented at national and international conferences and has undertaken research into service users' experience of mental health services and the physical health of people with schizophrenia. He has published numerous articles, a book on medication management and edited a book on psycho-social interventions.

Dr John Baker, MPhil, MSc, BNurs (Hons), RMN, CPN

John is a Lecturer in Mental Health Nursing in the School of Nursing, Midwifery and Social Work at the University of Manchester. He trained at the University of Manchester, qualifying as a mental health nurse in 1995, and has worked in a variety of inpatient settings, including acute and low secure rehabilitation. He has completed a number of postgraduate degrees, including his externally funded PhD (2007) 'Enhancing the use of "as required"/"extra" (PRN) medication within acute mental health settings' and an MPhil (2001), which led to the development of the Attitudes towards Acute Mental Health (ATAMH [33]). In 2003, he was appointed Lecturer in Mental Health Nursing. John continues to maintain good links with the NHS, supporting research in the clinical area and has published over 20 articles relating to mental health nursing with a focus on inpatient care and research methodology.

Professor Richard Gray PhD, MSc, BSc (Hons), RN, Dip HE, DLSHTM, FEANS

Richard is Professor of Nursing Research at the University of East Anglia in Norwich. He trained at King's College as a mental health nurse and at the London School of Hygiene and Tropical Medicine in public health. He was awarded his PhD in 2001 from King's College London and in the same year he was awarded a prestigious MRC research training fellowship. Until 2008 he was Head of the Section of Mental Health Nursing at the Institute of Psychiatry, King's College London. Richard has an international reputation for his clinical and academic work on medication adherence and patient choice and has published many articles and book chapters. He regularly presents at national and international conferences.

Contributors

Jenny Blackshaw for the past 3 years has been the lead nurse for medicines management at Manchester Mental Health and Social Care Trust. She qualified as a mental health nurse in 1992. Prior to this role she worked as a Community Psychiatric Nurse for 10 years in both primary and secondary mental health care settings. She has a keen interest in non-medical prescribing and its influence on medicines management. She has recently developed training packages for non-registered practitioners to assist with medicines administration and medicines competency assessments for registered mental health nurses.

Dr David Branford is the Chief Pharmacist of Derbyshire Mental Health Services NHS Trust. He has over 30 years' experience as a practising pharmacist, and over 25 years involvement with psychiatric practice. His PhD focused on antipsychotic drugs in learning disabilities. In 1984 he was appointed as teacher/practitioner at De Montfort University, Leicester and he established and managed the MSc in Psychiatric Pharmacy until 1999. He has many publications on issues related to the use of psychiatric medicines and services. He has clinical experience as part of multidisciplinary teams in the sub-specialities of learning disabilities, older peoples' psychiatry, forensic psychiatry and general psychiatry. He is co-chair of the National Pharmacy subgroup of New Ways of Working in Mental Health Pharmacy.

Dan Bressington is a Senior Lecturer in Mental Health at the Department of Social Work, Community and Mental Health, Canterbury Christ Church University. Dan has worked clinically both in the community and on inpatient units and has an interest in working with people with severe and enduring mental illness and their families. He has published work relating to medication management and adherence with treatment.

Petra Brown is currently working as the Chief Pharmacist and Joint Manager of the trusts effectiveness team for the Manchester Mental Health and Social Care Trust. The effectiveness team promotes evidence-based practice through appropriate use of treatments, audit and research being devolved into practice. She worked previously as a clinical pharmacist in mental health at South Manchester and has 12 years' experience working in mental health services. Areas of interest, research and publication over the years have focused on prescribing for treatment-resistant schizophrenia and Alzheimer's disease, and she has recently been involved in the production of a range of booklets for the dual diagnosis services.

Howard Chadwick is a Senior Lecturer in Mental Health at the School of Nursing in the Faculty of Health and Social Care Sciences at Kingston University and St George's London University. He is a Medication Management Trainer for the Section of Mental Health Nursing at the Institute of Psychiatry and is currently leading a study looking at issues concerned with implementing medication management skills and knowledge in practice. His clinical experience is working with people with severe and enduring mental illness. Educationally and academically, his interests include psychopharmacology, schizophrenia, psychosocial interventions for severe and enduring mental illness, and the implementation of evidence-based interventions and skills development.

Dr Rob Chaplin is a Consultant Psychiatrist who works with adults in a community mental health team and inpatient unit for adults who have severe mental health problems. He is an Honorary Research Fellow at the Royal College of Psychiatrists' Research and Training Unit, where he pursues his research interests in the therapeutic alliance, mental capacity, violence on inpatient units and learning disability, and is involved in a variety of quality improvement projects.

Dr Jennie Day is a Pharmacist who has carried out research on service users' perspectives of mental health medication for 17 years. She obtained a BSc in Pharmacy in 1988 from Sunderland Polytechnic, an MSc in 1990 (Manchester University), a PhD in 1995 (Clinical Psychology, University of Liverpool) and an MPH (Public Health) in 1999 (University of Liverpool). She has worked in various universities and mental health trusts and is currently Advanced Mental Health Pharmacist for the Five Boroughs Partnership Trust. Her research has included a variety of quantitative and qualitative methods and she developed the Liverpool University Neuroleptic Side Effect Rating Scale (LUNSERS) as part of her PhD.

Dr Joy Duxbury is a Divisional Leader for Mental Health at the University of Central Lancashire and heads the development of and provision for research and education in this field. She has conducted extensive research into the role of the service user in the delivery of care and shared perspectives on organisational, environmental, social and interventional issues. Accordingly, the bulk of her research work and publications has been on interventions that address medication management and patient aggression and violence. Joy continues to work collaboratively on a number of projects in these areas.

Janine Fletcher is a Lecturer at the University of Manchester and works on the Improving Access to Psychological Therapy programme. She is a mental health nurse with extensive experience in primary mental health care service delivery, development and research. She has worked as a therapist and manager in primary care since 1997. From 2002 to 2005 she worked as a primary care facilitator for the National Institute for Mental Health in England (NIMHE-NW) and was instrumental in the successful implementation of primary care graduate mental health workers in the north-west region. She is the author of the nationally acclaimed NIMHE commissioning guide for primary care. She has also been engaged in a wide range of research into the effectiveness of self-help interventions and has published widely in this field. Janine is also a trainer for a national skill-based suicide prevention programme (STORM).

Dr Michael Grierson has for the past 4 years been working in statutory mental health services, managing the development of a social inclusion service in Manchester. Prior to that he project managed the Recovery Education and Support Project at Having A Voice, a user-led voluntary organisation in East Manchester. His PhD was an action research study into the nature and uses of self-help within the Hearing Voices Network. In this regard, he was fortunate to be involved in the early years of a thriving national complex of hearing voices groups. Over the past 18 years or so he has learnt so much about recovery from this network.

Alison Hay for the past 3 years has been working as a Senior Lecturer at Staffordshire University. Prior to this she held a senior nursing position in an NHS trust in the West Midlands focusing upon quality improvement, non-medical prescribing and medicines management. Her clinical background is in adult community mental health nursing and she holds a specialist interest in severe and enduring mental health problems, family/carer issues and post-natal depression.

Steve Hemingway has been practising as a mental health nurse for over 20 years, working in acute inpatient, liaison psychiatry, brain injury rehabilitation and crisis/home treatment services. He has been a lecturer for 10 years at the Universities of Sheffield and Huddersfield. Psychopharmacological knowledge and medication management skills are something that he feels passionately that mental health nurses need to practise safely and competently. He has published widely on the area of mental health nurse prescribing (journals and book chapters) and is focusing his PhD study on medicines management implementation.

Steven Jones is a Senior Lecturer in continuing professional development (mental health) at Edge Hill University. His research interests include mental health law, homicide and complex clients with substance misuse issues. He is presently undertaking a PhD entitled 'Substance misuse and coercive treatments in withdrawal'. His clinical background includes adults with brain injuries, and severe and enduring mental health problems in criminal justice and forensic settings.

Dr Paul Lelliott is a Consultant Psychiatrist who is a member of a busy, multi-professional community assessment and treatment team in south-east London. He has also worked half-time as the director of the Royal College of Psychiatrists' Research and Training Unit since 1995. In this capacity he has led a range of national health services research projects and established the College Centre for Quality Improvement, which manages a programme of national quality improvement initiatives that involve many mental health care services in Great Britain and Ireland.

Peter Pratt is the Chief Pharmacist for Sheffield Care Trust and Rotherham Doncaster and South Humber (RDASH) NHS Mental Health Foundation Trust. He graduated from Portsmouth School of Pharmacy in 1977 and started to work as a specialist pharmacist in psychiatry in 1980. Appointed as Principal Pharmacist for mental health and community services, he subsequently became Chief Pharmacist for mental health services in Sheffield in 1994. Before taking on responsibility for RDASH he was also clinical director for substance misuse services in Sheffield. He has been involved in various national working groups relating to pharmacy and medicines in psychiatry, including New Ways of Working and the National Institute for Clinical Excellence clinical guideline development groups for Schizophrenia and Violence. In 1999, he was given the United Kingdom Psychiatric Pharmacy Group (UKPPG) chairman's award for outstanding contribution to pharmacy services in psychiatry.

Dr Alan Quirk is a Research Sociologist and Research Fellow at the Royal College of Psychiatrists' Research and Training Unit in London. He specialises in using qualitative methods to study communication in mental health care, and has a particular interest in understanding the obstacles to shared decision-making in psychiatric practice. Before this he worked at the Centre for Research on Drugs and Health Behaviour, Imperial College, where he worked on various qualitative studies, including a study of how methadone decisions are negotiated by staff and service users in drug dependency units.

Professor Clive Seale is a Professor of Medical Sociology, Queen Mary, University of London. Previously at Brunel University and Goldsmiths, he has interests in both medical sociology and social research methods. His interests have included end-of-life decision-making by doctors, interaction in healthcare settings, representations of health and illness in the mass media and on the internet, gender and the language of illness, and investigation of the experience and care of the terminally ill. His books include *Constructing Death* (Cambridge University Press, 1998), *The Quality of Qualitative Research* (Sage, 1999) *Media and Health* (Sage, 2003), *Researching Society and Culture* (Sage, 2004) and *Qualitative Research Practice* (co-edited with Gobo, Gubrium and Silverman; Sage, 2004).

Jim Turner is Mental Health Lead and Principal Lecturer in Mental Health at Sheffield Hallam University. He has been a mental health nurse since 1985. He has worked in a number of clinical settings as a staff nurse and manager. He is particularly interested in therapeutic interventions and medicines management.

Jacquie White is a Lecturer in Mental Health Nursing at the University of Hull and has been a mental health nurse for the last 21 years. She first became interested in medicines management when working as a research nurse in the late 1990s. Supported by a scholarship from the Florence Nightingale Foundation, she studied the role of the nurse in medication management on the acute unit for her first degree. She founded the Hull and East Riding medication management network in 2001 and the M62 Network in 2004. Both these networks continue to meet regularly to support members to implement and disseminate good medicines management practice. Currently, Jacquie is a leading role for medication management for both pre- and post-registration and non-medical prescribing courses. In 2006, she was awarded a University Teaching Fellowship in recognition of her medication management work.

Stuart Wix is a Forensic Nurse Consultant at Reaside Clinic, in the forensic directorate of Birmingham and Solihull Mental Health Trust, and took up this challenging post in July 2001. He was formerly a Forensic Community Psychiatric Nurse CPN team leader at Reaside Clinic. His interests include leading a 5-day medication management training programme, non-medical prescribing and research. He has an MA in Criminology from Keele University (1997) and is an honorary lecturer at the Department of Health Sciences at Birmingham University.

Preface

Medication has featured as the prominent treatment option in mental health care over the last 50 years. Despite the massive investment in developing these therapies, limited work has been conducted on the processes associated with the prescription and administration of medications. Indeed it is only in the last 10 years that clinicians and service users have begun to meaningfully discuss the options for treatment. This book is designed to help improve the meaningfulness of this process by providing clinicians with the knowledge required to not only just prescribe or administer psychotropic medications but engage in the whole process of medicines management.

The book is designed for a range of mental health professionals, practitioners and students and it is hoped that, regardless of current knowledge, it will offer something new. It provides the reader with access to some of the most up-to-date research and thinking in this area, and is written by a diverse range of experts, including mental health nurses, pharmacists, psychiatrists and researchers. In an effort to standardise meaning throughout the book several terms have been adopted. Firstly 'medicines management' has been adopted as term which describes the whole process. Secondly, 'service user' has been selected as a term which refers to people using mental health services; the authors feel this is a preferable option to patient or client.

The book is divided into two parts: the first provides underpinning knowledge on psychotropic medications and some of the potential interactions they have, and the second explores medicine management issues in clinical practice. This starts by exploring current policy and the perception of a service user towards medication and recovery. It describes the role of the prescriber and pharmacist before providing summaries of skills needed to meaningfully engage with, evaluate and solve problems associated with medications.

Part 1

An evidence base for medicines management

Introduction to medicines management

Neil Harris

Introduction

Psychotropic medication plays a pivotal role in treatment of many mental health problems (Appleby, 2005). In the case of psychotic disorders and dementia, medication fulfils a crucial role in treating the conditions; in other conditions such as anxiety and eating disorder, medication plays a more supplementary role to psychological interventions. The role that medication plays in these disorders changes along a continuum from managing acute episodes to maintaining stability and preventing relapse. Enabling a person to obtain the maximum benefit from the pharmacological aspects of their package of care has been subsumed under the name of 'medicines management'. This term, and the objectives that it encompasses, represents a complex and diverse set of processes that place the service user at the heart of the decision-making.

Medicines management consists of two interacting processes. Firstly, to enable the prescription of the most effective drug regimen to improve or maintain mental health whilst minimising adverse effects and, secondly, to enable the service user to become effective in managing his or her medication, maximising the benefits of being prescribed this optimum regimen. Key to the success of this work is the engagement of the service user in a genuine and trusting therapeutic alliance with the care team and, if appropriate, family and close friends. However, this is not a simple or straightforward process as attention to many factors and issues are required to establish an effective pharmacological intervention. It is hoped that this book will equip practitioners with some of the skills required to do this. This opening chapter will examine and explore these factors and issues and develop a coherent overview of medicines management.

The essential ingredient: the collaborative relationship

Psychotropic medications have an individual response; each person taking them can react differently to the same dose of a drug. It is crucial therefore, not only from an ethical point of view but from a clinical perspective that the taker has a central role in the process. There are important areas of practice that help people become involved in decisions about their medication. Evaluating treatment involves monitoring medication effects and changes in physical and mental health, which is facilitated by an atmosphere that encourages an ongoing interchange of information.

Care coordinators or key-workers take a lead role in coordinating the multi-disciplinary range of services and health care the service user receives. In certain circumstances, for example when working with a person with a serious mental illness or Alzheimer's disease (AD), a major part of this job is concerned with the management of medicines. A fundamental aspect of this role is in the development of the ongoing therapeutic relationship, developing a genuine and honest partnership in the planning of care and treatment, engaging in meaningful discussions about treatment options and alternatives, identifying and acting on areas of concern, and enabling people to take an active part in their treatment.

To achieve this essential relationship requires professionals to develop constructive and beneficial attitudes and beliefs. Central to this are the beliefs that service users have the capacity to recover, adapt and develop a meaningful, valued and quality life, despite the difficulties and distress they may suffer. This can only be achieved if service users are provided with time to develop their understanding and skills regarding medication, which will provide the relationship with a foundation that enables the service user to use medication to its maximum advantage.

A model of medication management

A modified version of Usher and Arthur's (1997) model (Figure 1.1) provides an overview of medicines management and represents both treatment effects and the role of the mental health practitioner.

The model views the process of treatment along two continua, the desired–undesired aspects of the treatment, and how this relates to the advocacy and empowerment roles of the practitioner. On the positive arm of the two continua, the practitioner's role relates to an empowered and informed service user. At the other end, a serious adverse effect of medication and ineffective or unsafe prescribing directs the practitioner to develop an advocacy role. The model provides a

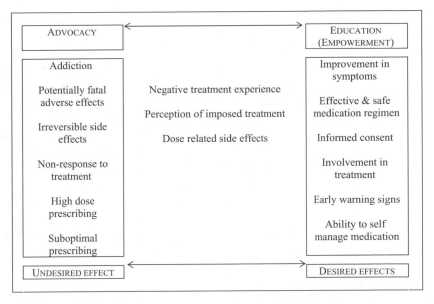

Figure 1.1 Model of medication management (modified). (From Usher, K. and Arthur, D. (1997) Nurses and Neuroleptic Medication: Applying theory to a working relationship with clients and their families. *Journal of Psychiatric and Mental Health Nursing*. Reproduced with permission of Wiley-Blackwell.)

simple overview of the roles undertaken in medicines management but also illustrates the complex and comprehensive nature of effective intervention. Medicines management work with the individual service user can focus on different, and possibly multiple, points, along these continua. Two clinical situations will now be explored to illustrate issues related to the advocacy and empowerment roles of mental health practitioners.

Example 1: Developing a safe and effective dosing regime

A common example of unsafe and ineffective practice can be found in the treatment of psychosis: polypharmacy. Polypharmacy is the practice of prescribing two or more antipsychotic drugs at the same time. This practice is continually discouraged and not recommended (Taylor et al., 2007; Joint Formulary Committee, 2008). The accumulative effect of combining two or more antipsychotics can result in high-dose prescribing and exposing the service user to multiple side-effect profiles. Many side effects are dose related and this practice not only increases the probability of the service user experiencing side effects but a wider range of side effects. It also increases the risk of cardiac arrhythmias, such as QT-prolongation and sudden cardiac death (Waddington et al., 1998; Taylor, 2003). Nevertheless the practice, which confers no benefit over the prescription of moderate doses of a single antipsychotic and has no formal evidence base, is widespread (Royal College of Psychiatrists, 2006). Polypharmacy and high doses are discussed in more detail in Chapter 13.

High doses and polypharmacy are difficult situations for the mental health practitioner to manage. The advocacy role would direct practice to enable the prescription of a safer regimen. Difficulties in this area can be addressed by collecting information useful in the prescribing process. By using a comprehensive assessment of mental state and side effects, taking a full medication history and undertaking discussions with the service user about treatment experiences, the practitioner can present the detailed information necessary for effective prescribing decisions.

The practitioner can make further recommendations:

- reductions in dosage, demonstrated to improve outcomes in some service users on high doses (Liberman et al., 1998; Suzuki et al., 2003),
- prescription of an alternative antipsychotic: many service users prescribed polypharmacy have not had an adequate trial with a single antipsychotic (Schumacher et al., 2003), or
- a trial of clozapine, as evidence suggests higher levels of polypharmacy in services which demonstrate a reduced use of clozapine (Chong et al., 2000; Purcell & Lewis, 2000).

These pharmacological suggestions are in addition to the psychological interventions for symptom management that may be put in place.

It has been noted that polypharmacy has a negative impact on service users' adherence to treatment (American Psychiatric Association, 1997). This situation can cause a difficult ethical dilemma as in these circumstances delivering interventions to increase treatment adherence may not be in the service user's best interest. This can result in conflicts between the prescribers and other practitioners. However, in areas of disagreement the Nursing Midwifery Council's position is clear: if the service user's interests are compromised by a proposed treatment, nurses are expected to advocate on their behalf to promote and safeguard their interests (UKCC, 1996, 1998).

In contrast to this situation, evidence suggests that service users treated for anxiety in primary care services may receive insufficient dose and duration of pharmacological treatment, leading to ineffective symptom relief. Management in this circumstance follows the same principles of developing information through assessment and discussion and using this as evidence to support recommendations made to the prescriber.

Example 2: Empowerment

The clinical example that develops the practitioner's role of empowerment is found in the care and treatment of people suffering from AD. Alzheimer's disease is a neurological disorder, which results in progressive deterioration in cognitive processes and behavioural problems. A relatively new pharmacological treatment has been developed from the cholinergic hypothesis (Davis & Maloney, 1976), which postulates that some cognitive problems experienced in AD are a result of a dysfunction in the cholinergic system. The aim of this type of medication, known as 'cholinesterase inhibitors', is described in more detail in Chapter 2. Their use has provided consistent results in delaying the deteriorating functioning of this condition (Evans et al., 2000).

Adams and Page (2000) provide a useful review of the implications for medicines management with these medications. Their partnership approach covers the duration of this pharmacological intervention from early intervention, through monitoring and finally to the discontinuation of treatment when benefits are no longer present. They support the practice of providing a full and honest disclosure of the advantages and limitations of treatment when seeking consent, particularly regarding the discontinuation of treatment, a difficult phase of the therapy. This process provides a platform for decision-making and planning early in the intervention. A crucial role of the management plan includes systematic monitoring of the benefits of medication and physical illness, which may compromise treatment. The involvement of the person and his/her family is an important aspect of this work. When evidence from monitoring indicates the treatment is no longer improving or maintaining the service user's levels of functioning, the treatment team then negotiates discontinuation. This is recognised as a painful and catastrophic time for the person and family, and is a situation that requires a sensitive and compassionate response as well as the need to develop care plans for the future.

Medicines management in this field highlights the empowering role of the practitioners: the need for complete and understandable information to enable service users and carers to take part in therapeutic discussions and form realistic treatment decisions. It is also important for the service users to be assessed for their capacity to consent to treatment and involved in the monitoring of symptoms and functioning. It must be noted that even though recent innovations in the care of AD employ an early intervention model, service users with mild to moderate AD have cognitive impairments, which may compromise their capacity to consent to treatment (Karlawish et al., 2005).

Key principles in medicines management

The following principles of practice are common to all areas of medicines management, irrespective of diagnosis or nature of pharmacological interventions.

Recovery

The concept of recovery in mental health has had many definitions. From a traditional medical perspective, recovery occurs when symptomatology is eliminated and the person returns to previous state of health and functioning, yet this clinical definition is now seen as inadequate to describe what recovery means to an individual. The effects of mental illness can impact on all aspects of a person's life, and recent descriptions have incorporated this idea. The concept of recovery has taken a meaning which reflects people's ability to engage in a process where they re-take control and responsibility over their lives, developing hope and optimism for the future, learn to adapt and maximise their strengths, and rebuild and reclaim their self-confidence and value in society (British Psychological Society, 2000; National Institute for Mental Health England, 2005; Rethink). Service users have identified the use of medication as a helpful strategy in moving towards recovery (Mental Health Foundation, 2000). A stated aim of medicines management is developing the person's self-efficacy in managing his/her pharmacological treatment. In this context, service users may decide on a variety of medication options. They may wish to titrate their medication against their subjective experience of illness/wellness. They may request work to develop a crisis medication plan against an assessment of their early warning signs. They may wish to try to become medication-free. These are areas where the practitioner can help minimise the risks through planning and support. The theme of recovery will be revisited throughout this book to highlight the areas where medication and the role of the practitioner can enhance this process.

Adherence and consent

Non-adherence to medication has been cited as a major problem across all healthcare groups, especially when used for long-term chronic illness management, where about half the medication prescribed is not taken (Haynes et al., 1996). Sufferers of schizophrenia are five times more likely to experience a relapse if they decide to discontinue their medication (Robinson et al., 1999). Subsequent relapses lead to increased recovery times, poor long-term outcomes (Kane et al., 1998) and reduced levels of functioning (Hogarty et al., 1991), presenting a range of negative consequences for the person and his/her family. For some people non-adherence can also result in depression. This carries the risk of an accumulation of medication in the person's home, providing a ready means of acting on suicidal ideas.

The circumstances that result in non-adherence stem from two root causes. It can be unintentional, the result of forgetting or poor administration routines. In these situations interventions can be put in place to attend to identified difficulties. Intentional, also called 'covert', non-adherence, is where the service user decides not to take all or a proportion of the prescription and, commonly, does not tell the care team about this decision. Another aspect of non-adherence is where a 'supervising' relative holds a negative appraisal of the medication and withholds or administers doses below that prescribed to the relative (Bollini et al., 2004).

There is an interface between the concepts of adherence and consent; they are both concerned with taking prescribed medication. Engaging the service user in the process of consent is a fundamental right. It is also an important aspect in developing the therapeutic relationship and enables people to feel in control of their health care and demonstrate their personal responsibility in directing treatment (Harris et al., 2002).

This can be a difficult and sometimes controversial procedure, given the complexity of medication-related information that service users need to review in order to be considered 'informed', where cognitive difficulties may hamper the successful learning of material or the person feels pressured to accept the treatment and the issue of capacity to make a valid decision. Medication is usually prescribed to a service user when the condition is in its acute phase. In some situations medication may be prescribed and administered in the service users' 'best interest' as their mental state renders them incapable of providing valid consent. However, at the earliest opportunity the process must begin and be viewed as a process rather than an event: an ongoing collaborative practice that guides and underpins treatment goals. In circumstances where the process of consent has been valid, that the service user is informed, free to choose and has mental capacity, practitioners need to be aware of the inclination to provide further 'persuasion' if the service user decides not to follow medical advice (Brabbins et al., 1996). The practitioner needs to be cognisant when applying strategies to improve adherence that these strategies are not seen as pressure to conform to the prescribed regimen.

In circumstances where a person perceives a threat to his or her personal freedom, a mindset can develop which motivates the person to respond in a way which aims to restore and assert his or her autonomy – a construct known as 'psychological reactance' (Brehm, 1966). In a study that explored the attitudes of people with schizophrenia who were prone to feel in this way, those who held the view that taking medication was a threat to their freedom of choice were more likely to have been non-adherent in the past (Moore et al., 2000). Providing service users with an opportunity to talk about medication, through the process of consent, can result in increased self-confidence and self-efficacy as they become more informed and involved in making treatment decisions and this can generalise to taking control of other aspects of their lives (Rogers et al., 2003).

A recent conceptualisation of the relationship between the service user's acceptance of medication and the practitioner's advice has been termed 'concordance'. Concordance is not a replacement for either compliance or adherence; it is a different concept, which shifts the focus from the service user's behaviour to the quality of a partnership of shared decision-making. It is a process where agreement regarding the prescription and taking of medication is reached by discussion within an alliance in health care. These issues will be developed in later chapters.

The evidence base for medication management

Two main intervention areas have been the targets for research in medicines management. Some researchers have developed programmes that have sought to enable service users to become skilled in the self-management of their treatment. A more recent development has seen research that has involved teaching mental health professionals to deliver medicines management packages. There follows a limited review of the evidence supporting this work.

Teaching service users to self-manage medication

It has been established that providing information to service users about mental illness and treatment does not result in non-adherence. Detailed education programmes were delivered to service users with schizophrenia and included information about serious side effects such as tardive dyskinesia (TD), without reduction in adherence rates (MacPherson et al., 1996; Chaplin & Kent, 1998). They also noted that informing people about TD late in treatment carried the risk of creating alarm or anger in service users or their relatives. Providing a full range of information in an accessible and honest way, whilst encouraging the service user to ask questions, is an essential skill of medication management and facilitates collaborative decision-making and consent.

There are a number of studies where practitioners have sought to develop a collaborative relationship with service users through the use of self-care packages which have included education, medication administration skills training and cognitive–behavioural strategies. Boczkowski et al. (1985) and Eckman et al. (1992) used educational programmes and took a behavioural orientation which incorporated tailoring administration to service users' daily routines and the use of self-monitoring for medication effects and early warning signs. Calendars and workbooks were used to maintain a focus on the targets of intervention. In both studies services users' knowledge and adherence improved, although methodological problems weaken these findings.

'Compliance therapy' (Kemp et al., 1996) evaluated an intervention for psychotic in-patient service users. Grounded in motivational interviewing (Miller and Rollnick, 1991) and cognitive–behavioural techniques, participants received twice weekly sessions lasting 20–60 minutes over a period of between 4 and 6 weeks. Significant improvements in insight, compliance and attitude towards medication were measured, which were sustained at 6-month follow-up. Booster sessions were given at 3, 6 and 12 months and improvements were maintained at 18 months (Kemp et al., 1998). Methodological considerations cited by the authors include the high attrition rate of 35%, the observer-rated method of assessing compliance, outcome measures were rated by the research psychiatrist who was not blind to the treatment status resulting in potential observer bias, and the lack of statistical power. In a study which replicated compliance therapy in a group of service users diagnosed with schizophrenia (O'Donnell et al., 2003), the authors concluded that the intervention did not confer a major advantage over counselling for compliance, symptoms, attitude to treatment, insight, functioning or quality of life.

Randell et al. (2002) propose two strategies for improving adherence: a compliance intervention (likened to Kemp et al., 1996) and an alliance intervention. The alliance intervention provided a framework for problem formulation, medication history, self-evaluation of treatment and issues regarding communicating with professionals. Alliance therapy developed from research exploring clients' experiences in taking medication (Day & Bentall, 1996; Rogers et al., 1998). Service users are regarded as rational consumers who are able to evaluate medication for themselves and that 'appropriate adherence' will result if the medication is having a positive effect. Both of these interventions consist of 8–12 half-hour sessions. The two strategies can be seen to fall along a continuum, with the compliance intervention being more suitable for service users who are positive about the medication but lack information, and alliance therapy, indicated for service users with a more negative attitude towards medication or medical care. It was clarified that in practice service users' needs may sit somewhere between these positions and the intervention package is constructed that addresses their individual positions. Only single-case studies are available for these interventions but show promising initial results.

Teaching medication management to practitioners

In a cluster randomised controlled trial, Gray et al. (2004) developed a medicines management training package and taught it to 60 community mental health nurses (CMHNs). The educational programme lasted 80 hours and was based on the *Compliance Therapy Manual* (Kemp et al., 1997). Community mental health nurses were taught to deliver the intervention to two services users from their caseload who had a diagnosis of schizophrenia and were considered to have poor adherence. Following training, CMHNs demonstrated significant improvements in their knowledge and skills in compliance therapy (Gray et al., 2003). Significant improvements were seen in the psychopathology and attitude to treatment of service users. Methodological considerations cited by the authors include the high 26% attrition rate, and possible biases introduced as a result of the use of self-report and clinician ratings, and the selection of the study's service users by their CMHNs.

Another medication management training programme was developed and evaluated by Harris et al. (2008). A 10-day training programme sought to enable 28 community mental health practitioners (CMHP), mainly nurses but with occupational therapists and social workers, to deliver a collaboration-based medicines management programme. The training addressed the components involved in achieving an effective medication regimen and self-management strategies. Issues related to adherence and achieving adherence were confined to methods that can be undertaken by 'moderately experienced clinicians who lack specific training in cognitive-behavioural skills' (Randell et al., 2002). Community mental health practitioners worked with four of their service users, who had a diagnosis of schizophrenia, over a 9-month period. Service users whose CMHPs undertook the training made significant improvements in their symptoms and perception of their involvement in treatment.

Service users can become active participants in developing effective illness management programmes; with increasing responsibility for treatment, they are the pivotal change agent for personal recovery. A number of essential ingredients and interventions have been identified which enable this process to occur. However, it must be understood that a consequence of increasing the self-efficacy and empowerment that these programmes confer may not result in increased adherence but when adherence is increased is it based on the service user's choice.

The skills of the workforce

All members of the care team have responsibilities in managing service users' medication. *The Ten Essential Shared Capabilities* are areas of aptitude considered to be a requirement of all mental health workers, and these represent basic principles that underpin positive practice (Hope, 2004). This framework of competencies, developed by service users, carers and practitioners, provides a blueprint to achieve best practice and includes core and specialist skills. The four key areas identified are ethical practice, knowledge, an understanding of the process of care and expertise in effective interventions. These capabilities have a direct relevance to the skills used in medication management and are reviewed here emphasising these areas.

Working in partnership

This develops the focus of collaboration in care, engaging not only service users and their families in the process of management but those involved in the delivery of care, enabling clear and effective lines of communication and establishing clear understanding regarding the function of medication management. Service users and their families can have different views on the need and duration of treatment (Bollini et al., 2004), which can result in tension or coercion, emphasising the need for an approach that involves the family unit in information sharing and decision-making.

Respecting diversity

This is having the ability to deliver interventions which takes full account of the diverse nature of service users in terms of age, disability and gender, and demonstrating respect for their culture, spirituality and sexuality. Issues relating to race and culture are particularly relevant.

> 'Black and minority ethnic patients have worse access to, experience of, and worse outcomes from mental health services than the white majority population. In other words there is discrimination – direct or indirect – in mental health services'
>
> Speech by Rosie Winterton, Minister of State for Health Services: Race and Mental Health, Tackling Inequalities Conference, 8 March 2005

The Sainsbury Centre for Mental Health (2002) reports on the negative experiences of black people in relation to the prescription and administration of medication. Black service users receive higher doses of psychotropic medication, and administration was seen to be coercive and punitive. Fear of professional power compromises the service users' right to become involved in their treatment decisions or question professional decisions regarding medication, whose attitude they consider to be paternalistic and condescending.

Practising ethically
Inherent in the mental health nurses' central accountability to the service user is the recognition of the service users' rights (UKCC, 1996, 1998): the right to take an active and informed role in their medication-related treatment decisions, the right to a safe and effective drug regimen, and the opportunity to consent, or not, to treatment. Promoting these rights against conflicting professional viewpoints is a difficult responsibility. Practising ethically also involves working with the service user's aspirations, for example of becoming medication free and taking an honest, non-judgemental and neutral stance to medication-related issues.

Challenging inequality
People can experience feelings of stigma from being prescribed and taking psychotropic medication (Sirey et al., 2001; Dinos et al., 2004). Furthermore, the side effects of medication can compromise a person's social and vocational networks, for example Boumans et al. (1994) found that the presence of orofacial dyskinesia had a negative effect in a work-related interview process. Mental health workers need to be mindful of these consequences when developing treatment choices.

Promoting recovery
Recovery from mental illness is an individualised and personal journey that is dependent on a variety of factors, central to which is empowerment and self-determination. The attitudes and interaction style of mental health practitioners in this context has the aim of generating hope and an appreciation that developing a medication strategy which the person finds beneficial may need a long-term perspective requiring a realistic, flexible and responsive mental health service.

Identifying people's strengths and needs
Enabling service users to become effective in managing their mental health and developing an understanding of the role that medication plays in this process depends on working with the person's strengths and also his or her assets and supports. Skilled and timely assessments can identify areas that further empower service users to control their health care and can include the development of skills to negotiate treatment changes or finding more detailed information.

Providing service user centred care

Service user opinions regarding the place of medication in their mental health management can show wide variation dependent on the effectiveness of the medication, the benefit the drugs confer and the person's health beliefs. An additional dimension in this area is the extent to which a person wishes to be involved in his or her health care; from full involvement in the decision-making process to those who would prefer to leave the process to members of the care team (Hendrick, 2000). Short- and long-term goals are dependent on the viewpoint the person takes along these continua. Assessment plays an important role in this process, providing people with objective feedback in areas where little progress may be perceived and in the development of further targeted goals and care plans.

Making a difference

The skills and interventions that enable service users to evaluate and develop skills in medication self-management have a wide evidence base. There are key skills, a range of strategies and interventions that are available to engage the person in developing a dialogue that facilitates the service user's understanding and decision-making. These strategies will be discussed in a later chapter but include looking at a person's beliefs about medication, using timelines to explore past events and future aspirations, their attitude to taking or not taking medication, evaluating the advantages and disadvantages of medication, and problem solving. Using the services user's experience of what treatments work and what treatments should be avoided, advanced directives can be utilised in times of crisis to direct interventions when a service user may lack capacity to communicate his or her treatment wishes.

Promoting safety and positive risk taking

Being honest with service users about not only the positive aspects of pharmacological treatment but also the negative, especially the most serious adverse effects, is a crucial part of enabling self-management and an important part in developing the therapeutic relationship. For a number of people the positive aspects of treatment are limited and the experience of side effects outweighs the positive effects. Furthermore, for some people suffering from serious mental health problems, the prospect of living the rest of their lives taking medication is not a tenable situation. Many people may wish to try maintaining their health and lifestyle drug-free. Service users need to feel able to express this wish to mental health professionals and be supported both practically in terms of, for example, formulating a discontinuation plan, providing information, alternative methods of symptom management and the development of an early warning plan. Practitioners need to provide emotional support that demonstrates an empathic understanding for their decision. Service users may decide to independently and covertly discontinue their medication. The approach supported here is based on the premise that if a service user makes this decision, it is in the service user's interest if family members and care services know about it. Again, the crucial factor in enabling people to feel comfortable in sharing this information is the relationship they have with those people involved in the care process.

Personal development and learning

The continuous flow of evidence concerning the efficacy of pharmacological interventions, new drugs and interventions regarding management, require mental health practitioners to be proactive in maintaining their knowledge and skills. Practitioners also need to be able to reflect on their practice and values in dynamic and changing mental health services. The role of supervision in the development and maintaining of new skills and practice has been emphasised (Bradshaw, 2002; Clarke, 2004). A definition provided by 'Vision for the future' (Department of Health (DH), 1993) sits well in the medicines management framework:

> '. . . a formal process of professional support and learning which enables individual practitioners to develop knowledge and competence, assume responsibility for their own practice and enhance consumer protection and safety of care in complex clinical situations. It is central to the process of learning and to the expansion of the scope of practice and should be seen a means of encouraging self-assessment and analytical and reflective skills.'

> DH (1993)

Supervision for medicines management should function on a number of levels, developing practitioners' knowledge base by utilising a problem-solving approach focused on their caseload and reflective practice to address changing levels of competency in intervention areas, ethical and relationship issues. This process can be seen as a conscious and purposeful strategy to explore experience and learn from it (Getcliffe, 1996). The arrangements for developing supervision systems need to be context driven, making maximum use of available resources.

New ways of prescribing

Recent policy developments have enabled the introduction of new ways to prescribe medication, for example non-medical prescribing and patient group directions. Non-medical supplementary prescribing was introduced in 2003 and has been defined by the DH (2005) as:

> *'a voluntary prescribing partnership between an independent prescriber (doctor) and supplementary prescriber (nurse or pharmacist) to implement an agreed service user specific clinical management plan with the service user's agreement.'*

In May 2006, the DH further extended the role of non-medical prescribers by introducing independent non-medical prescribing:

> *'. . . Prescribing by a practitioner (e.g. doctor, dentist, nurse, pharmacist) responsible and accountable for the assessment of patients with undiagnosed or diagnosed conditions, and for decisions about the clinical management required, including prescribing.'*
>
> *DH (2006)*

and patient group directions:

> *'. . . written instructions to enable registered nurses to supply and administer a specified medication to a group of service users who may not be individually identified before treatment.'*
>
> *DH (2005)*

These developments represents a major innovation in the way nurses work and it is expected that this new modernisation in the way services are delivered will not only make better use of the knowledge and skills of nurses but will allow for more timely and effective medication changes and administration, and increase the service users' treatment choices. Two factors will be crucial to the safe and effective development of this new way of working:

i.   The nurse prescriber's knowledge and skills in medicines management and a commitment to continuous professional development together with a supportive infrastructure and resources to develop and improve practice;

ii. The establishment of clear professional and Trust strategies and policies, supported by key individuals and monitored through robust clinical governance structures.

Conclusion

Medicines management is a complex and difficult process requiring the practitioner and service user to engage in a dialogue across a number of inter-related aims. Practitioners need to develop and adjust their role with individual service users in light of changing circumstances: service users' abilities and skills in medication management, the effectiveness of the regimen prescribed and the condition and severity of the person's mental health experience. The foundation of effective management lies in the development of a genuine and trusting collaborative therapeutic relationship, evolved through the process of consent. If the service user's perception of services is positive – non-coercive, positive relationships with the care team, a regimen with minimal adverse effects and involvement in treatment decisions – service users are more prepared to accept treatment (Day et al., 2005). Sometimes the collaborative therapeutic relationship is difficult to achieve. Symptoms, experience with services and health beliefs can contribute to the failure to engage the service user. In these circumstances a long-term perspective and empathic attitude can mitigate against these situations.

Practitioners need to develop a wide range of knowledge and skills, as well as a positive attitude, regarding the opinions and capabilities of service users in the process of making maximum use of pharmacological intervention. This book is aimed at informing and guiding practitioners in developing relationships and applying interventions that enable service users to use a medication regimen that they find helpful in managing the distressing experiences and remaining well.

References

Adams, T. & Page, S. (2000) New pharmacological treatments for Alzheimer's disease: implications for dementia care nursing. *Journal of Advanced Nursing,* **31**, 1183–1188.

American Psychiatric Association (1997) Practice guidelines for the treatment of patients with schizophrenia. *American Journal of Psychiatry,* **154**, 1–63.

Appleby, L. (2005) Forward. In: Department of Health (ed.) *Improving Mental Health Services by Extending the Role Prescribing and Supplying Medication.* HMSO, London.

Boczkowski, J.A., Zeichner, A. & De Santo, N. (1985) Neuroleptic compliance amongst chronic schizophrenic outpatients: an intervention outcome report. *Journal of Consulting and Clinical Psychology,* **53**, 666–671.

Bollini, P., Tibaldi, G., Testa, C. & Munizza, C. (2004) Understanding treatment adherence in affective disorders; a qualitative study. *Journal of Psychiatric and Mental Health Nursing,* **11**, 668–674.

Boumans, C.E., de Mooij, K.J., Koch, P.A.M., van't Hof, M.A. & Zitman, F.G. (1994) Is the social acceptability of psychiatric patients decreased by orofacial dyskinesia. *Schizophrenia Bulletin,* **20**(2), 339–344.

Brabbins, C., Butler, J. & Bentall, R. (1996) Consent to neuroleptic medication for schizophrenia: clinical, ethical and legal issues. *British Journal of Psychiatry,* **168**, 540–544.

Bradshaw, T. (2002) Training and supervision in psychosocial interventions for people with schizophrenia. In: Harris, N., Willimas, S. & Bradshaw, T. (eds) *Psychosocial Interventions for People with Schizophrenia*. Palgrave MacMillan, Basingstoke.

Brehm, J.W. (1966) *A Theory of Psychological Reactance*. Academic Press, New York.

British Psychological Society (2000) *Recent Advances in the Understanding of Mental Illness and Psychotic Experiences*. British Psychological Society, London.

Chaplin, R. & Kent, A. (1998) Informing patients about tardive dyskinesia. *British Journal of Psychiatry*, **172**, 78–81.

Chong, S.A., Remington, G.J. & Bezchlibnyk-Butler, K.Z. (2000) Effect of clozapine on polypharmacy. *Psychiatric Services*, **51**, 250–252.

Clarke, S. (2004) *Acute Inpatient Mental Health Care: Education, Training & Continuing Professional Development For All*. National Institute for Mental Health in England and Sainsbury Centre for Mental Health, London.

Davis, P. & Maloney, A.J.F. (1976) Selective loss of central cholinergic neurones in Alzheimer's disease. *Lancet*, **310**, 1403.

Day, J., Bentall, R., Roberts, C., et al. (2005) Attitude toward antipsychotic medication: the impact of clinical variables and relationships with health professionals. *Archives of General Psychiatry*, **62**, 717–724.

Day, J.C. & Bentall, R.P. (1996) Schizophrenia patients' experience of neuroleptic medication: a Q-methodological investigation. *Acta Psychiatrica Scandinavica*, **93**, 397–402.

Department of Health (1993) *Vision for the Future: The Nursing, Midwifery and Health Visiting Contribution to Health and Health Care*. HMSO, London.

Department of Health (2005) *Improving Mental Health Services by Extending the Role of Nurses in Prescribing and Supplying Medication: Good Practice Guide*. HMSO, London.

Department of Health (2006) *Improving Patients' Access to Medicines: A Guide to Implementing Nurse and Pharmacist Independent Prescribing within the NHS in England*. HMSO, London.

Dinos, S., Stevens, S., Serfaty, M., Weich, S. & King, M. (2004) Stigma: the feelings of 46 people with mental illness. *British Journal of Psychiatry*, **184**, 176–181.

Eckman, T., Wirshing, W., Marder, S., et al. (1992) Technique for training schizophrenic patients in illness self-management; a controlled trial. *American Journal of Psychiatry*, **149**(11), 1549–1554.

Evans, M., Ellis, A., Watson, D. & Chowdhury, T. (2000) Sustained cognitive improvement following treatment of Alzheimer's disease *International Journal of Geriatric Psychiatry*, **15**, 50–53.

Getcliffe, K. (1996) An examination of the use of reflection in the assessment of practice for undergraduate nursing students. *International Journal of Nursing Studies*, **4**, 361–374.

Gray, R., Wykes, T. & Gourney, K. (2003) The effect of medication management training on community mental health nurse's clinical skills. *International Journal of Nursing Studies,* **40**, 163–169.

Gray, R., Wykes, T., Edmonds, M., Leese, M. & Gournay, K. (2004) Effect of a medication management training package for nurses on clinical outcomes for patients with schizophrenia. *British Journal of Psychiatry,* **185**, 157–162.

Harris, N., Lovell, K., Day, J. & Roberts, C. (2008) An evaluation of a medication management training programme for community mental health professionals; service user level outcomes A cluster randomised controlled trial doi:10.1016/j.ijnurstu.200810.010.

Harris, N., Lovell, K. & Day, J. (2002) Consent and long-term neuroleptic treatment. *Journal of Psychiatric and Mental Health Nursing,* **9**, 475–482.

Haynes, R.B., McKibbon, A. & Kanani, R. (1996) Systematic review of randomised trials of interventions to assist patients to follow prescriptions for medications. *Lancet* **348**, 3836.

Hendrick, J. (2000) *Law and Ethics in Nursing and Health Care.* Stanley Thornes, Cheltenham.

Hogarty, G.E., Anderson, C.M., Reiss, D.J., Korn-Blith, S.J., Greenwalk, D.P. & Ulrich, R.F. (1991) Family psychoeducation social skills training and maintenance chemotherapy in the aftercare treatment of schizophrenia II. Two year effects of a controlled study on relapse and adjustment. *Archives of General Psychiatry,* **48**, 340–347.

Hope R. (2004) *The Ten Essential Shared Capabilities – A Framework for the Whole of the Mental Health Workforce.* HMSO, London.

Joint Formulary Committee (2008) *British National Formulary.* British Medical Association and Royal Pharmaceutical Society of Great Britain, London.

Kane, J.M., Aguglia, E., Altamura, A.C., Gutierrez, J.L.A., Brunello, N. & Fleishhacker, W.W. (1998) Guidelines for depot antipsychotic treatment in schizophrenia. *European Psychopharmacology,* **8**, 55–66.

Karlawish, J.H.T., Casarett, D.J., James, B.D., Xie, S.X. & Kim, S.Y.H. (2005) The ability of persons with Alzheimer disease (AD) to make a decision about taking an AD treatment. *Neurology,* **64**, 1514–1519.

Kemp, R., Heyward, P. & David, A. (1997) *Compliance Therapy Manua.,* Bethlam and Maudsley NHS Trust, London.

Kemp, R., Heyward, P., Applewaite, G., Everitt, B. & David, A. (1996) Compliance therapy in psychotic patients: a randomised controlled trial. *British Medical Journal,* **312**, 345–349.

Kemp, R., Kirov, G., Everitt, B., Heyward, P. & David, A. (1998) A randomised controlled trial of compliance therapy: 18 month follow up. *British Journal of Psychiatry,* **172**, 413–419.

Liberman, R., Marder, S., Marshall, B.D., Mintz, J. & Kuehnel, T. (1998) Biobehavioural therapy: interactions between pharmacotherapy and behaviour therapy in schizophrenia. In: Wykes, T., Tarrier, N. & Lewis, S. (eds) *Outcome and Innovation in Psychological Treatment of Schizophrenia.* Wiley, Chichester.

MacPherson, R., Jerrom, B. & Hughes, A. (1996) A controlled study of education about treatment in schizophrenia. *British Journal of Psychiatry*, **168**, 709–717.

Mental Health Foundation (2000) *Strategies for Living*, Mental Health Foundation, London.

Miller, W.R. & Rollnick, S. (1991) *Motivational Interviewing: Preparing People to Change*. Guilford Press, New York.

Moore, A., Sellwood, B. & Stirling, J. (2000) Compliance and psychological reactance in schizophrenia. *British Journal of Clinical Psychology*, **39**, 287–296.

National Institute for Mental Health England (2005) *Guiding Statement on Recovery*. National Institute for Mental Health England, London.

O'Donnell, C., Donohoe, G., Sharkey, L., et al. (2003) Compliance therapy: a randomised controlled trial in schizophrenia. *British Medical Journal*, **327** (doi:10.1136/bmj.327.7419.0).

Purcell, H. & Lewis, S. (2000) Postcode prescribing in psychiatry: Clozapine in an English county. *Psychiatric Bulletin*, **24**, 420–422.

Randell, F., Wood, P., Day, J.C., Bentall, R., Roger, A. & Healy, D. (2002) Enhancing appropriate adherence with neuroleptic medication: two contrasting approaches. In: Morrison, A.P. (ed.) *A Casebook of Cognitive Therapy for Psychosis*. Brunner-Routledge, New York.

Rethink. *A Brief Introduction to the Recovery Approach*. London. www.rethink. org/recovery/index.htm (accessed January 2008).

Robinson, D., Woerner, M.G., Alvir, J., et al. (1999) Predictors of relapse following response from first episode of schizophrenia or schizoaffective disorder. *Archives of General Psychiatry*, **56**, 241–247.

Rogers, A., Day, J., Randall, F. & Bentall, R. (2003) Patients' understanding and participation in a trial designed to improve the management of antipsychotic medication. A qualitative study. *Social Psychiatry and Psychiatric Epidemiology*, **38**, 720–727.

Rogers, A., Day, J.C., Williams, B., et al. (1998) The meaning and management of neuroleptic medication: A study of patients with a diagnosis of schizophrenia. *Social Science and Medicine*, **47**, 1313–1323.

Royal College of Psychiatrists (2006) *Consensus Statement on High-Dose Antipsychotic Medication*. Royal College of Psychiatrists, London.

Schumacher, J., Makela, E. & Griffin, H. (2003) Multiple antipsychotic medication prescribing patterns. *Annals of Pharmacotherapy*, **37**, 951–955.

Sirey J.A., Bruce M.L., Alexopoulos G.S., Perlick D.A., Friedman S.J., & Myers B.S. (2001) Perceived stigma and patient-rated severity of illness as predictors of antidepressant drug adherence. *Psychiatric Services*, **52**, 1615–1620.

Suzuki, T., Uchida, H., Tanaka, K., et al. (2003) Reducing dose of antipsychotic medications for those treated with high dose antipsychotic polypharmacy: an open study of dose reduction for chronic schizophrenia. *International Clinical Psychopharmacology*, **18**, 323–329.

Taylor, D., Paton, C. & Kerwin, R. (2007) *The Maudsley Prescribing Guidelines 2006–2007*. Taylor and Francis Group, London.

Taylor, D.M. (2003) Antipsychotics and QT prolongation. *Acta Psychiatrica Scandinavica*, **107**, 85–95.

The Sainsbury Centre for Mental Health (2002) *Breaking the Circles of Fear*. The Sainsbury Centre for Mental Health, London.

UKCC (1996) *Guidelines for Professional Practice*. United Kingdom Central Council for Nursing, Midwifery and Health Visiting, London.

UKCC (1998) *Guidelines For Mental Health and Learning Disability Nursing*. United Kingdom Central Council for Nursing, Midwifery and Health Visiting, London.

Usher, K. & Arthur, D. (1997) Nurses and neuroleptic medication; applying theory to a working relationship with clients and their families. *Journal of Psychiatric and Mental Health Nursing*, **4**, 117–123.

Waddington, J.L., Youssef, H.A. & Kinsella, A. (1998) Mortality in schizophrenia: antipsychotic polypharmacy and absence of adjunctive anticholinergics over the course of a 10-year prospective study. *British Journal of Psychiatry*, **173**, 325–329.

Psychotropic medications

Howard Chadwick and Dan Bressington

Introduction

Mental health nurses play a vital role in the process of managing psychiatric medication. In order to maintain the safety of service users, mental health nurses should aim to maximise the potential benefits of treatment and minimise any associated adverse effects. A good understanding of psychopharmacology will provide a platform on which the healthcare professional can build confidence and skills when helping clients to manage their medication.

In this chapter we explore the most commonly used groups of psychotropic medication. Each group and sub-class of psychotropic drug is considered in terms of mechanism of action, effectiveness, adverse effects and possible drug interactions. The key medication management issues that relate to each class of drug are also summarised and the final part of the chapter examines the most dangerous of possible adverse outcomes. The analysis of each group of medications is not intended to be exhaustive and we encourage the reader to access additional sources of information that provide comprehensive details of individual drugs.

Antipsychotics

Antipsychotic medication, as the name implies, is used to treat symptoms of psychosis. Antipsychotics were also known as neuroleptics and in times past were referred to, somewhat misleadingly, as major tranquilisers. Chlorpromazine, the first of the antipsychotics, was introduced in 1952 and was the first effective treatment for psychosis. The impact of this cannot be underestimated and it led Holmes to observe that:

> *'Almost overnight, psychiatric wards were transformed from "snake pits" where patients lived in strait jackets and were largely out of control to places of relative calm and order.'*

Holmes (1994), p. 332

Research and development led to a group of related drugs, the phenothiazines, and other drugs which acted in similar ways but were chemically distinct, such as the butyrephenones (e.g. haloperidol and droperidol) and thioxanthenes (e.g. zuclopenthixol). Collectively these may be considered the typical or first generation antipsychotics. Subsequently a second generation of antipsychotics was developed, which became known as the atypical antipsychotics, as they have a notably different side-effect profile from the typical group. The first to be launched was clozapine, followed by others such as risperidone, olanzapine and quetiapine. Recently, with the introduction of aripiprazole, it may be said that a third generation of antipsychotics has emerged; these drugs have a different mechanism of action to both the typical and atypical drugs.

Although there are many large-scale trials of antipsychotics which allow us to make broad statements about their effects, individual responses remain idiosyncratic. Often, finding the drug that best suits a person is a matter of trial and error. However, broad guidance for treatment is contained in *Schizophrenia: Full National Clinical Guideline on Core Interventions in Primary and Secondary Care* (National Collaborating Centre for Mental Health, 2003).

Treatment adherence with antipsychotics is a major clinical issue impacting on areas such as safety, relapse and long-term prognosis. Kikkert et al. (2006) explored factors that influenced treatment adherence with antipsychotics in a European, multi-centre concept mapping study. Results showed that the single most important factor for service users was whether or not the treatment was effective. The second most important factor was side-effect self-management. Understanding the pharmacology of antipsychotics enables clinicians to assist clients in addressing these factors.

Typical antipsychotics

Mechanism of action

Extensive research was undertaken into the mechanisms of action of typical antipsychotics. This has led to the development of a range of theories regarding the pathology of psychosis. Over time, it became clear that it was the ability to act as a dopamine antagonist that produced the clinically desirable effect, and by 1993 McKay and McKenna were confident in stating:

> *'In short, that the antipsychotic effects of neuroleptic drugs is a consequence of the ability to block dopamine receptors must be regarded as established beyond reasonable doubt.'*
>
> *McKay & McKenna (1993)*

However, dopamine blockade serves merely to ameliorate the positive symptoms of psychosis, such as auditory hallucinations, delusions and paranoia, which often persist at a residual, albeit more tolerable, level. Positive symptom reduction is thought to derive from the blockade of dopamine D2 receptors in the meso-limbic system. The therapeutic effect takes time to develop and full response may take several weeks. Side effects, however, emerge immediately. In an acute phase, rapid acting adjunctive treatment such as a benzodiazepine to reduce distress and ensure safety should be considered.

Evidence of effectiveness

There is now more than 50 years of clinical experience treating psychosis with typical antipsychotics and an equivalent quantity of research. Typical antipsychotics are all equally effective at treating the positive symptoms of psychosis and overall approximately 80% of people will respond to treatment. Detailed summaries of the efficacy of individual drugs are available as systematic reviews from the Cochrane Collaboration. Typical antipsychotics do not improve negative symptoms and may indeed exacerbate them (Stahl, 2000).

Side effects

Typical antipsychotics are sometimes classified, in the *British National Formulary* for example, by their side-effect profile. This is dependent on their propensity to act not only as an antagonist at dopamine D2 receptors but at other dopamine receptors and other types of receptors such as alpha-1 adrenaline, H1 histamine and M1 acetylcholine receptors. These are predictable from the receptor-binding profile of the drug and usually dose-dependent. Normal therapeutic ranges provide for maximum desired response. Prescribing in higher doses often merely leads to increased side effects.

Dopaminergic side effects

While dopamine D2 blockade in the meso-limbic pathway produces the desired symptom relief, three other pathways, the meso-cortical, nigro-striatal and tuberoinfundibular, all use D2 receptors and are also blockaded. This leads to a series of side effects dependent on the function of each pathway.

Meso-cortical blockade has been implicated in the exacerbation of cognitive impairment and negative symptoms. It is thought that the meso-cortical pathway may already have lowered dopaminergic activity in those suffering from schizophrenia, and treatment serves to compound this problem.

Nigro-striatal blockade leads to a range of movement disorders, including dystonias, pseudo-parkinsonian symptoms, akathisia and tardive dsykinesia. These are referred to as extrapyramidal side effects (EPSE). These are often found to be the most distressing and debilitating symptoms among people taking the drug and have been identified as one of the causes of non-concordance.

Acute dystonic reactions, such as an oculogyric crisis, where the eyes roll back in the head, or torticollis, where there is contraction of the neck muscles, are due to muscle spasm and can be life-threatening. Treatment is usually intra-muscular administration of an anticholinergic, which provides rapid relief. Younger, treatment-naïve people are more likely to develop an acute dystonic reaction.

Pseudo-parkinsonism (tremor, rigidity, bradykinesia and bradyphenia) can also be alleviated by the use of anticholinergics, reduction in dose or use of an atypical antipsychotic. This is due to the reciprocal nature of dopamine and acetylcholine in the nigro-striatal pathway. Dopamine antagonism produces a relative excess of cholinergic activity. By inhibiting cholinergic activity the ratio between dopaminergic and cholinergic activity is restored to some extent, thus reducing the side effects.

Another distressing side effect in this group is akathesia, a subjective sense of inner restlessness. It is associated with irritability from a behavioural perspective and in extreme, aggression and suicide. There is debate regarding treatment efficacy for akathesia with anticholinergics favoured in the UK and low-dose propanalol in the USA, although there appears little to choose between them (Cunningham-Owens, 1999).

A debilitating and irreversible movement disorder associated with long-term treatment is tardive dyskinesia (TD). It is characterised by facial contortions, particularly of the mouth and tongue, and uncontrolled limb movements. Its cause remains rather unclear but appears to be a response to prolonged D2 antagonism in the nigro-striatal pathway whereby the receptors up-regulate or become supersensitive to combat the blockade, which leads to hyperactivity. Approximately 5% of people maintained on typical antipsychotics will develop TD every year (Stahl, 2000).

Tuberoinfundibular pathway dopamine blockade leads to a rise in the level of the hormone prolactin. This pathway normally prevents the release of prolactin and when its action is impaired, prolactin levels rise, leading to hyperprolactinaemia. This causes a range of side effects, including galactorrhoea (milk production), gynaecomastia (breast tissue development), amenorrhoea (menstrual disturbances) and sexual dysfunction.

Alpha-1 adrenergic
Alpha-1 adrenaline antagonism leads to cardiovascular side effects such as orthostatic hypotension, electrocardiogram (ECG) changes, tachycardia and drowsiness.

H1 histaminergic
H1 histamine antagonism is responsible for drowsiness and weight gain.

M1 cholinergic
M1 acetylcholine receptor blockade produces a range of side effects such as dry mouth, blurred vision, constipation and cognitive impairment. However, drugs with a strong anticholinergic profile have a lower propensity to induce EPSEs due to self-regulating the dopamine : acetylcholine activity ratio in the nigro-striatal pathway.

The varying propensity of phenothiazines to induce these side effects led them to be classified in three groups (Table 2.1). All other typical antipsychotics, including typical depot preparations, have a profile similar to Group 3.

Unpredictable side effects
For some side effects it is not possible to predict occurrence or severity from a drug's pharmacology. The most serious condition is neuroleptic malignant syndrome (NMS). This is characterised by high temperature, muscle rigidity, confusion and labile blood pressure (Caroff and Mann, 1993). Two indicative pathology results are a raised creatinine phos-

Table 2.1   Side-effect profiles of typical antipsychotic medication

	Extrapyramidal side effects	Anticholinergic	Sedation
Group 1 (e.g. chlorpromazine)	Moderate	Moderate	High
Group 2 (e.g. pericyazine)	Moderate	High	Moderate
Group 3 (e.g. trifluoperazine)	High	Moderate	Moderate

phokinase (CPK) level and leucocytosis. Early recognition of the condition is important as it is potentially fatal and requires specialised interventions. All antipsychotics may induce it, although trifluoperazine and haloperidol seem to present a higher risk. It is most likely to occur in the first 2 weeks of treatment, although estimates of incidence vary from 0.5 to 2.2% of cases. There is evidence to suggest that a diagnosis of bipolar affective disorder and administration by injection significantly increases the risk (Hermesh et al., 1992).

A further serious side effect is delay of cardiac repolarisation shown by a prolonged QTc interval on ECG recordings. This is discussed in the danger zones section of this chapter. Antipsychotics may also cause a range of other side effects that are less common, such as blood dyscrasias, including agranulocytosis and leucopenia, rashes, jaundice and photosensitisation.

Interactions

It should be stressed that all co-prescribing should be checked for potential interactions. The co-prescribing of antipsychotics, which induce QTc prolongation with tricyclic antidepressants, increases the risk. Similarly, the use of anxiolytics and hypnotics has an additive sedative effect. Antipsychotics also antagonise the anti-convulsant effect of carbamazepine and valproate, thereby lowering the seizure threshold. The interactions with non-prescribed medication are discussed in Chapter 3.

Atypical antipsychotics

The term 'atypical' is applied to the second generation of antipsychotics owing to their reduced propensity to cause EPSEs. The first of this group was clozapine, which was first synthesised in 1958 (Hippius, 1999). After initial launch in the 1970s it was withdrawn because of the recognition of previously unidentified and potentially fatal but rare side effects. It was re-launched with a restricted licence in the UK in 1990, and was followed by other drugs.

Mechanism of action

Like the typical antipsychotics, atypicals reduce positive symptoms through dopamine D2 antagonism in the meso-limbic pathway. They are equally as effective as typical antipsychotics with the possible exception of clozapine, which is a fairly weak D2 antagonist. As a group they may be viewed as dopamine D2 and serotonin 5-HT2A antagonists but in other respects they are quite individual. Clozapine is the most complex, acting as an antagonist at no fewer than seven serotonin and four dopamine receptor subtypes. How these actions combine remains unclear, although evidence shows that it is superior in efficacy to typical antipsychotics (Wahlbeck et al., 1999) and helps a proportion of those resistant to conventional treatment (Verhoeven et al., 1992). It is suggested that other atypicals may have some beneficial effect on negative symptoms but the evidence remains rather equivocal (Sanders & Mossman, 1999; Gardner et al., 2005). The hypothesis regarding both efficacy for negative symptoms and the low incidence of EPSE concerns the atypicals' serotonin 5-HT2A receptor antagonism. Serotonin has extensive influence on dopamine activity but this is not consistent between the dopamine pathways. In the meso-cortical pathway where dopaminergic deficiency is thought to relate to negative symptoms, 5-HT2A antagonism causes an increase in dopamine activity. In the nigro-striatal pathway serotonin inhibits dopamine release. Antagonism at 5-HT2A enhances dopamine release, allowing for greater competition at D2 receptor sites between the drug and dopamine and so reducing the proportion of D2 antagonised receptors and reducing side effects (Stahl, 2000).

Evidence of effectiveness

Extensive research has compared not only atypicals with typical antipsychotics but with each other (Geddes et al., 2000). It appears that there is little difference in symptom response between the atypicals and typicals or between them, with the exception of clozapine (Wahlbeck et al., 1999; Geddes et al., 2000; Gardner et al., 2005). Clozapine has been shown to help somewhere between 40 and 70% of people deemed treatment-resistant. For those who have a poor response to clozapine, various augmentation strategies have been tried but evidence concerning their efficacy remains equivocal (Kontaxakis et al., 2005; Remington et al., 2005).

Atypical antipsychotics have a low propensity to induce EPSEs but this does not mean to say that they never cause them (Margolese et al., 2005; Mendhekar, 2005; Ghaemi et al., 2006). Risperidone is the most likely to induce movement disorders and this is dose related. Atypicals are far from side-effect free but they produce unwanted effects that differ from typicals. While the side-effect profile alters in individuals and drugs, there are some characteristic unwanted results of treatment with this group. Weight gain causes considerable problems, being both a health risk, which may be associated with the onset of diabetes, and also a major adherence issue. This is variable across the group, with clozapine and olanzapine producing the greatest weight gain, and a higher incidence of diabetes (Cunningham-Owens, 1999; Mir and Taylor, 2001), and ziprasidone the least (Ananth et al., 2004; Gardner et al., 2005). Individual drugs have particular problems. Probably the best known is the risk of agranulocytosis with clozapine. A potentially fatal condition, this affects the immune system, lowering white cell counts and impairing an individual's ability to fight infection. Regular blood tests are needed to monitor the possible development of this condition. Clozapine may also cause hypersalivation, which although not danger-ous, is highly debilitating socially. Clozapine can prove highly sedating to the point where it affects an individual's quality of life. Similarly, amisulpiride, which has a moderately low side-effect profile overall, is more likely to raise prolactin levels than other atypicals. There have also been concerns about some atypicals inducing prolonged QTc inter-vals. This caused sertindole to be withdrawn from the market, although it is now undergoing further clinical trials. Ultimately the profile for an individual is an idiosyncratic expression of the interaction of the person and the drug. Minimising side effects and increasing tolerability are often a matter of trial and error. However, there is no doubt that the reduction of the occurrence of EPSEs has improved the tolerability of atypicals over typicals and has led to the National Institute of Clinical Excellence (NICE) guidelines recommending the use of atypicals as first-line treatment (National Institute of Clinical Excellence, 2002).

Interactions

All co-prescribing should be approached with caution and interactions checked. Of note is carbamazepine's ability to increase the metabolism of atypicals, which may result in the need for a higher dose to maintain therapeutic levels. The reverse is true of some of the selective serotonin re-uptake inhibitor (SSRI) antidepressants, particularly fluoxetine, which can increase plasma levels and require a reduced dose of atypi-cals. The co-prescribing of typical and atypical antipsychotics (poly-pharmacy) should be avoided as it negates the benefits of the newer drugs.

Third-generation antipsychotics

The development of antipsychotics has been inextricably linked with hypotheses about the pathology of schizophrenia. The pharmacology of the drugs has informed our understanding of the pathways and processes involved in both desired and unwanted effects. This in turn has pointed the way to develop new compounds that improve efficacy and tolerability. The first of the third generation of antipsychotics to enter clinical practice is aripiprazole. Others are in various stages of clinical trials. They differ from previous antipsychotics in having a different mechanism of action.

Mechanism of action

Aripiprazole is a partial dopamine agonist with a strong affinity to D2 receptors. Its action allows it to reduce dopaminergic activity where there is too much (meso-limbic pathway) and increase it where there is too little (meso-cortical pathway). It is also a partial agonist of 5-HT1A receptors and an antagonist of 5-HT2A. It only shows a weak affinity for H1 histamine, alpha-1 adrenergic and cholinergic receptors (Davies et al., 2004; Hirose and Kikuchi, 2005; Kontaxakis et al., 2005). Theoretically it should address both positive and negative symptoms while reducing the possibility of sedation, weight gain, hyperprolactinaemia and movement disorders. This should improve tolerability.

Evidence of effectiveness

A systematic review of clinical trials to date (El-Sayeh & Morganti, 2006) has demonstrated that the efficacy of aripiprazole is similar to other atypical antipsychotics. At present there is little evidence available to demonstrate that it has superior treatment response or tolerability.

The pharmacology of aripiprazole suggests that many familiar side effects will be avoided, most commonly reported are akathisia, sleepiness and nausea, particularly in the early stages of treatment. There are also some reports of the occurrence of movement disorders (Fleischhacker, 2005; Desarkar et al., 2006; Sharma & Sorrell, 2006; Zacher & Hatchett, 2006; Ziegenbein et al., 2006). As yet it is not possible to determine any long-term effects of treatment because, despite its increasing clinical use, aripiprazole has still only been available for a relatively short time (Stahl, 2000).

Interactions

Aripiprazole plasma levels are prone to alteration by the co-prescribing of a variety of drugs such as carbamazepine, fluoxetine, paroxetine, phenytoin and St John's wort. Although not strictly an interaction, attention should also be drawn to potential problems initiating aripiprazole, particularly during an acute phase. As it is non-sedating and potentially activating, consideration should be given to adjunctive treatment with a benzodiazepine or a sedating antihistamine such as promethazine. Key points regarding antipsychotic medicines can be found in Box 2.1.

Box 2.1 Antipsychotics – Key points

- All antipsychotics are effective at treating positive symptoms.
- Atypicals may help negative symptoms.
- Only clozapine has been consistently shown to help some people who are treatment-resistant.
- Side effects are a common reason why people stop their medication.
- High doses usually only increase side effects.
- Minimising side effects aids concordance.
- Co-prescribing typicals and atypicals negates the benefits of atypicals.
- Giving accurate information supports informed decisions.

Mood stabilisers

Bipolar disorder affects approximately 1% of the global population. It is characterised by variations in mood from mania through to depression. It usually first appears in adolescence and is equally distributed between men and women. There are three main pharmacological treatment options available for bipolar disorder: lithium salts, anti-convulsants and antipsychotics.

Lithium

Mechanisms of action

Lithium remains the first-line treatment option after some 50 years of clinical use. Despite this wealth of experience and the fact that it is a simple molecule, its mechanisms of action remain poorly understood. More detail is becoming available concerning its ability to affect gene expression in the neuron (Lenox & Wang, 2003) and the mechanisms involved may help explain the time lag between commencement of therapy and improvement. It is also known that lithium alters the permeability of the cell membrane to a number of cations including Na^+, Ca^{2+} and Mg^{2+}, and so affects changes in neuronal polarity and neurotransmitter release (Gurvich & Klein, 2002).

Evidence of effectiveness

Lithium has been shown to be effective in the treatment and prophy-laxis of both bipolar and unipolar mood disorders (Burgess et al., 2001; Goodwin and Geddes, 2003). It has been shown to prevent suicide and deliberate self-harm (Cipriani et al., 2005). However, it has been found that it is most effective in classic manic-depressive cases and less so in atypical presentations (Kleindienst & Greil, 2003). In these cases, alternative monotherapy or combination therapy should be considered.

Side effects

Lithium has a narrow therapeutic range. Monitoring of blood serum levels is necessary to ensure both therapeutic efficacy and avoidance of toxicity. The desired level lies between 0.4 and 1.0 mmol/l. The side effects encountered at therapeutic levels include a range of gastro-intestinal disturbances such as nausea, vomiting and diarrhoea. Also common is fine tremor and increased thirst. Lithium is given as a salt, either carbonate or citrate, and this increases thirst. Weight gain is a common problem with lithium treatment and oedema is sometimes present. Lithium also affects thyroid function and can cause hypothy-roidism. This is characterised by fatigue, weakness, weight gain, hair loss, poor memory, muscle cramps and aches, decreased libido, dry rough skin and cold intolerance. Regular renal and thyroid function tests should be undertaken to monitor for these side effects and it is important that people are made aware of the signs to aid early recognition. Levels above 1.5 mmol/l may be fatal. Signs of toxicity include confusion, convulsions, ataxia, dysarthria, nystagmus, tremor and renal impairment. If signs of toxicity are present, treatment should cease and serum levels determined. Appropriate action should be taken to reduce the serum level. Urgent action is required for levels of 2.0 mmol/l and above. Both polyuria and polydipsia can occur and instances of lithium-induced nephrogenic diabetes insipidus have been reported (Baylis & Heath, 1978; De Soto et al., 1985; Kosten & Forrest, 1986; Illowsky & Kirch, 1988; Eustatia-Rutten et al., 2001). Lithium toxicity is discussed in further detail later in this chapter.

Interactions

Lithium has a range of interactions and co-prescribing should always be checked for adverse effects. Diuretics reduce lithium excretion as do angiotensin converting enzyme (ACE) inhibitors and angiotensin II receptor antagonists and so raise serum levels. Lithium increases the risk of EPSEs with phenothiazines, haloperidol, sulpiride and clozapine. There is an increased risk of toxicity with tricyclic antidepressants and an increased risk of ventricular arrhythmias with sertindole. All these issues are under the control of the prescriber but of particular note is the probable ability of non-steroidal anti-inflammatories (NSAIDs) to raise serum levels. This is problematic as drugs such as ibuprofen are available over the counter.

Anti-convulsants

Mechanisms of action

This group includes carbamazepine, valproate and lamotrigine. Like lithium, the mechanism of action of anti-convulsants is poorly understood. What is known is that they also alter the permeability of ion channels in the cell membrane and influence the inhibitory neurotransmitter gamma-aminobutyric acid (GABA). Their effects on GABA include enhancing its synthesis and release, while also inhibiting breakdown and re-uptake. They may also enhance its action at receptor sites. In addition, it is thought they may also reduce the release of glutamate, the universal excitatory neurotransmitter. This combination of effects can be summarised as not only putting on the brakes by enhancing GABAergic activity but also taking the foot off the accelerator by impeding glutamatergic activity (Wolf et al., 1988; Stahl, 2000).

Evidence of effectiveness

Carbamazepine has been shown to be effective, and may be superior in cases of rapid cycling bipolar disorder, but otherwise the anti-convulsants seem equally efficacious. Whether they are as effective as lithium, particularly regarding prophylaxis, remains equivocal (Macritchie et al., 2001, 2003).

Side effects

Carbamazepine was derived from tricyclic antidepressants and shares some of the side effects of that group, particularly anticholinergic ones. These include drowsiness, dizziness, sexual dysfunction, constipation and visual disturbances. It can also cause arrhythmias, blood dyscrasias and skin problems. A generalised mild rash is common in early treatment but usually disappears. If it worsens or other symptoms are evident, treatment should be withdrawn. More serious and rare is Stevens–Johnson syndrome, the first indications of which are usually non-specific symptoms such as cough, headache and fever. A rash develops, usually on the face and neck, which then blisters particularly around the mucous membranes. Eventually the skin may peel away, as can hair and nails. This condition is potentially fatal due to the risk of infection. Carbamazepine may also impair liver function and this should be regularly monitored. Valproate also causes a range of gastrointestinal disturbances such as nausea and diarrhoea but also causes an increase in appetite and weight gain. Valproate may also induce transient hair loss and liver dysfunction. Lamotrigine has a similar side-effect profile but is notable for causing skin reactions, including Stevens–Johnson syndrome. The anti-convulsants may also cause foetal abnormalities such as neural tube defects. It is important that information and support about this issue is provided for women and their partners where appropriate.

Interactions

Carbamazepine induces the action of CYP450 enzymes and so can reduce the level of many other drugs, including tricyclic antidepressants and clozapine. Conversely, fluoxetine, fluvoxamine, erythromycin and isoniazid increase carbamazepine levels. Valproate has fewer interactions but there is an increased risk of neutropenia when used with olanzapine.

Antipsychotics

The use of antipsychotics as adjunctive treatment to mood stabilisers during manic episodes has a long history of clinical use. What has become apparent is that some atypical antipsychotics may have a more prolonged role to play in both the treatment and prophylaxis of bipolar disorder (Chengappa et al., 2004; Vieta & Goikolea, 2005; Marken & Pies, 2006; Nguyen & Guthrie, 2006; Pini et al., 2006). In the UK both olanzapine and quetiapine are approved for treating mania. Key points regarding mood stabilisers can be found in Box 2.2.

Box 2.2   Mood stabilisers – key points

- Many of these drugs have serious side effects, which require careful monitoring.
- People need information to monitor themselves.
- There is an increasing choice of drugs available that should enable better tailoring of treatment to individual needs and preference.

Antidepressants

Depression is a very common mental health problem and antidepressants are prescribed widely in many care settings. According to the NICE guidelines (National Institute of Clinical Excellence, 2004) all individuals at risk for depression should be screened and, if a decision is made to prescribe medication, the drug of choice should be an SSRI. Psychotropic medication should be part of a package of care that includes psychosocial interventions such as cognitive behavioural therapy (CBT), self-help techniques and problem solving. Antidepressants appear to be of little value (and therefore should not be prescribed) for people experiencing mild depression.

Individuals experiencing a depressive episode that requires drug treatment should be experiencing one or more of the following symptoms in addition to low mood: changes in appetite/weight/sleep, low energy, feelings of guilt/worthlessness or suicidal ideation. It is clinically very useful to obtain a measurement of depression at baseline and then periodically to provide a measure of change.

Mechanisms of action and effectiveness

There are a variety of explanations as to why drugs can help to relieve depression. It appears that depression may be caused by a lack of noradrenalin or serotonin or both. All classes of antidepressants act at the synapse in varying ways to increase the action of these neurotransmitters. There are three groups of typical antidepressants: tricyclic antidepressants (TCAs), SSRIs and monoamine oxidase inhibitors (MAOIs). In addition to these there are a variety of novel or atypical antidepressants. Animal experiments have demonstrated how the therapeutic benefits of these drugs are related to the effects they have on neurotransmitters.

Tricyclic antidepressants are the original antidepressants (e.g. amitriptyline) and seem to work by preventing some of the re-uptake of serotonin and noradrenaline at the pre-synaptic neurone, making more available to deliver messages over the synapse. These medicines are effective but not very selective in terms of how much, and which, neurotransmitter is increased. The only exception to this is the more modern reboxetine, which appears to be more selective in inhibiting noradrenaline re-uptake.

Monoamine oxidase inhibitors (e.g. phenelzine) also increase the monoamines serotonin and noradrenaline, but this is achieved by inhibiting the enzyme that breaks down the neurotransmitters in the presynaptic neurones and the glial cells around the synapse. For some unknown reason MAOIs appear to work a little quicker than other classes of antidepressants. A more recent MAOI (moclobemide) works in the same way but only temporarily inhibits the enzyme monoamine oxidase and as a result is sometimes called a reversible monoamine oxidase inhibitor (RIMA).

Selective serotonin re-uptake inhibitors are the most commonly prescribed antidepressants (e.g. fluoxetine and paroxetine). They work in a similar way to the TCAs but are very selective in terms of mainly inhibiting the re-uptake of serotonin and by having less effect on a whole range of other receptors that result in unwanted effects.

Atypical antidepressants (e.g. venlafaxine) are classed as such because they cannot be grouped under the three typical groups owing to the differences in mechanisms of action. Venlafaxine, for example, is called a serotonin noradrenaline re-uptake inhibitor (SNRI) because it is more selective in terms of inhibiting the re-uptake of noradrenaline and serotonin.

The theories about mechanisms of action are rather simplistic and do not adequately explain why the delayed onset of therapeutic benefit of these medicines occurs. The acute action of the drugs at the neurotransmitters is relatively quick but the clinical benefits are not seen at the same time. One of the many theories is that there is a delayed change of neurotransmission in both the pre- and post-synapses; this change may relate to the way the synapses adapt to the presence of the drug (i.e. by possibly increasing the amount of receptors at the post-synaptic cleft) (Vaswani et al., 2003). The clinical benefit of antidepressants may also relate to the relationship between serotonin and dopamine, but again this mechanism is not well understood.

The differences in effectiveness of improving mood in the wide variety of antidepressants is negligible (Simon, 2002). The main differences in the effects seen in clinical practice relate to which other receptors are acted upon and the half-life of the drug concerned. Clinical experience suggests individual symptoms vary between different people and similarly the most effective drug will vary accordingly.

The Maudsley Prescribing Guidelines (Taylor et al., 2007) reviews literature on the minimum recognised effective doses required for antidepressants. The differences in an individual's ability to metabolise the medicine account for the need for increased doses in some people. In terms of the commonly used antidepressants:

- the dose for TCAs is unclear although at least 75–100 mg/day
- fluoxetine, citalopram and paroxetine require a minimum of 20 mg/day
- sertraline and fluvoxamine need to be at least 50 mg/day
- venlafaxine requires a dose of at least 75 mg/day and the moclobomide dose should be a minimum of 300 mg/day.

Side effects and drug interactions

The clinical efficacy of all antidepressants is very similar but it is the side-effect profiles of these drugs that really distinguish them from each other. These adverse effects will directly influence the acceptability of the drug to the individual (Ashton et al., 2005). The side effects of antidepressants differ because of the differences in the way they work on a variety of receptors. The mechanism of side-effect action is better understood than the mechanism of action of clinical benefit.

Tricyclic antidepressants commonly cause sedation, postural hypotension, tachycardia, marked anticholinergic effects, weight gain and are cardiotoxic. The weight gain and sedation probably relate to histamine (H1) antagonism. The blockade of adrenergic receptors appears to cause changes in cardiovascular function, and anticholinergic effects are related to the blockade of muscarinic receptors. Sexual dysfunction is also reported in TCAs; this probably relates to increased noradrenaline and serotonin (Brill, 2004). All the adverse effects can influence acceptability to the client but the most worrying of all the unwanted effects in terms of mortality is cardiotoxicity. If taken in overdose, TCAs are very likely to cause death; this is the reason why NICE recommends the use of SSRIs, which are much safer in terms of toxic effects in overdose. The major interactions of TCAs include other antidepressants (which can raise plasma levels of TCAs, causing toxicity), alcohol (increased sedation and toxicity) and antimuscarinics (increased anticholinergic effects). Caution is also advised if an antipsychotic is co-prescribed, owing to an additive effect of increased adverse effects.

Monoamine oxidase inhibitors can cause similar unwanted effects as the TCAs but may additionally result in headaches, insomnia and leucopenia. The adrenergic-related side effects are more marked in the MAOIs (resulting in a decreased heart rate); however they are less cardiotoxic than TCAs. Classic MAOIs are better tolerated than TCAs but can result in hypertensive crisis if food is eaten containing tyramine. This reaction and the subsequent dietary restrictions is probably why MAOIs are not widely prescribed. Moclobemide is less likely to cause this interaction owing to its reversible nature of action.

Selective serotonin reuptake inhibitors are widely associated with nausea, vomiting, sexual dysfunction, insomnia, agitation and discontinuation syndrome. Hyponatraemia (low blood sodium levels) can also be seen rarely; however, there is a possibility of all antidepressants causing this, particularly in older people. The side effects of SSRIs are most likely to arise from the effects on noradrenaline and serotonin. Because SSRIs are metabolised by an array of P450 liver enzymes, interactions may occur (they can alter plasma levels of other drugs). This potentially serious interaction is examined later on in the chapter.

Selective serotonin reuptake inhibitors are far less cardiotoxic than TCAs and also do not tend to cause sedation, weight gain and anticholinergic effects.

Sexual dysfunction can occur with antidepressants. Measuring this is complicated by the fact that similar sexual problems are often seen in people who are depressed but have not yet taken medication. Around 40–50% of people report reduced libido and 15–20% of people report orgasm problems prior to diagnosis (Kennedy et al., 1999). The prevalence of sexual dysfunction associated with antidepressants varies between the different classes of antidepressants but it appears that SSRIs are more commonly associated with libido and orgasm problems, which are reported in 60–70% of cases. Tricyclic antidepressants cause similar problems in around 30% of people and in MAOIs the figure is around 40% (Taylor et al., 2007). Sexual side effects cause great distress and as a result are associated with non-adherence to treatment. Ashton et al. (2005) surveyed 750 service users taking antidepressants and found that after weight gain, sexual dysfunction was most commonly cited as being the reason for non-adherence. Service users and professionals can find talking about sexual matters difficult. However, as it is very important that sexual dysfunction is identified, a number of standardised measures have been developed to measure sexual dysfunction, and clinical experience has found that the Arizona Sexual Experiences Scale (McGahuey et al., 2000) is useful in approaching the subject and in providing a standardised measure of problems. *The Maudsley Prescribing Guidelines* (Taylor et al., 2007) suggest switching to a drug less likely to cause problems, if appropriate, stopping the treatment, and a variety of drug treatments such as sildenafil, that should be managed by a sexual dysfunction specialist.

As a general rule, different groups of antidepressants should not be prescribed concurrently owing to the risk of serotonin syndrome, possible elevated plasma levels and additive adverse effects. Serotonin syndrome is a potentially fatal condition caused by the toxic effects of excess serotonin at the pre- and post-synaptic neurones (Gilman, 2006). The symptoms of serotonin syndrome are usually present in the following order: restlessness, diaphoresis, tremor, shivers, myoclonus, confusion, convulsions and eventually death. The most likely drug combinations to cause this serious problem are SSRIs and MAOIs (Leonard & Richelson, 2003).

Discontinuation syndrome

Discontinuation syndrome has received a lot of media attention and has been mistakenly labelled as withdrawal symptoms, suggesting that antidepressants are physiologically addictive. This is not the case as they are not associated with physical tolerance and craving. The National Institute of Clinical Excellence (2004) advises that all service users who are prescribed antidepressants should be aware that discontinuation symptoms can occur if the drug is stopped, if doses are missed, and sometimes when the drug is reduced. These symptoms are generally mild but on occasion they can be severe and distressing and are more likely if the medication is stopped abruptly. As some of the symptoms experienced can be similar to the symptoms of depression, they may be perceived as a relapse of the illness. All classes of antidepressants can cause discontinuation symptoms. The mechanism of action of discontinuation syndrome is thought to be related to a rebound effect of action at receptors that were previously blocked (Lejoyeux et al., 1993). Tricyclic antidepressants and SSRIs cause very similar discontinuation symptoms such as flu-like symptoms, insomnia, vivid dreams, irritability and occasionally movement disorders. Monoamine oxidase inhibitors do not appear to cause flu-like symptoms but they can cause other effects similar to SSRIs/TCAs, and agitation, speech problems and occasionally hallucinations/delusions (Haddad & Anderson, 2007). The half-lives of the different antidepressants are closely related to the severity of discontinuation symptoms. Drugs with short half-lives (e.g. paroxetine, amitriptyline and venlafaxine) can cause symptoms if the drug dose is missed, whilst this is less likely for drugs with longer half-lives (e.g. fluoxetine). In fact *The Maudsley Prescribing Guidelines* (Taylor et al., 2007) recommend that fluoxetine can be used to help manage discontinuation symptoms, owing to its longer half-life. They also recommend that any discontinuation should be carried out over a minimum of 4 weeks to reduce the chance of symptoms being severe.

St John's wort

St John's wort is a widely used herbal medicine that is both prescribed and bought over the counter for use as an antidepressant. It is a derivative of the plant *Hypericum perforatum*, but usually contains many other compounds. The exact compound responsible for the antidepressant effect is unknown and the mechanism of action is not well understood but could relate to its action on serotonin, noradrenaline and dopamine. To complicate matters further the levels of different compounds found in different preparations vary dramatically, making research on efficacy difficult (Mennin & Gobbi, 2004).

The National Institute of Clinical Excellence (2004) state that it is likely that St John's wort may have some efficacy in mild depression but should not be prescribed or used, owing to the lack of evidence and that it is an unlicensed herbal remedy. A systematic review of the evidence by Linde et al. (2005) concluded that specific extracts of St. John's wort may have some efficacy in treating mild to moderate depression, although the data are not fully convincing. The known side effects of St John's wort include: dry mouth, nausea, constipation, fatigue, headache and restlessness. Service users should always be asked if they are taking St John's wort (or any other non-prescribed treatment) as it increases the action of P450 enzymes that can result in a lowering of plasma levels of some prescribed drugs. Due to its serotonergic action it can cause serotonin syndrome if taken with other prescribed antidepressants. The seriousness of possible interactions should be reinforced to patients who may view herbal remedies as being inherently harmless (McGarry et al., 2006; Taylor et al., 2007). Key points regarding antidepressant medicines can be found in Box 2.3.

Box 2.3   Antidepressant – key points

- Antidepressants should not be prescribed for mild depression.
- Selective serotonin re-uptake inhibitors are recommended as first line treatment and are safer.
- Discontinuation syndrome is likely; clients should be advised and antidepressants should be slowly stopped over at least 4 weeks.
- Antidepressants are most effective if given with psychosocial treatment.
- Antidepressants take several weeks to work.
- The desired and adverse effects of antidepressants should be monitored using standardised rating scales.

Anti-anxiety medicines

Anxiolytics are widely prescribed in primary and secondary mental health services despite the NICE guidelines (National Institute for Clinical Excellence, 2004) highlighting that the preferred treatments for anxiety are psychosocial treatment or self-help approaches based on CBT principles. In clinical practice, drug interventions are often necessary due to the difficulties accessing psychosocial treatments. Where medication is prescribed NICE recommend that the first-line treatment should be an SSRI antidepressant. If benzodiazepines are to be used they should be prescribed for a limited period (2–4 weeks) and that they should be used for emergency management only (not for obsessive compulsive disorder (OCD) or post-traumatic stress disorder (PTSD)).

When attempting to manage anxiety it is always worth considering if it is associated with a co-morbid mental health problem, for example drug/alcohol use, depression or psychosis. The recommended drug treatment for anxiety disorders depends upon which type of anxiety is diagnosed. Anxiety disorders can be classed under the following groups: generalised anxiety disorder (GAD), panic disorder, social phobia, OCD and PTSD.

Antidepressants

The issues surrounding antidepressants have already been discussed and we refer the reader to the previous section in terms of side effects and interactions. If prescribed an SSRI, the service user should be informed that there is a possibility of anxiety symptoms becoming more pronounced before the therapeutic effect is achieved. The mechanism of action of antidepressants in anxiety management is as equally baffling as the mechanism of action for depression and, owing to the delayed onset of therapeutic action, these drugs have no place in the acute management of anxiety. The mechanism of action could be related to the complex relationship between changes in neurotransmission of serotonin, noradrenaline, dopamine and some GABA receptors (Leonard & Richelson, 2003).

Benzodiazepines

Benzodiazepines (BDZs) (e.g. diazepam, lorazepam, clonazepam) are widely prescribed for a variety of stress-related illnesses. However, their use is sometimes unjustified (Joint Formulary Committee, 2008). They are also sometimes used for insomnia, alcohol withdrawal management, muscle relaxation, emergency seizure control and rapid tranquilisation.

Mechanism of action

The way BDZs work is more fully understood than most psychotropic drugs. Throughout the central nervous system (CNS) a naturally occurring transmitter molecule called GABA exists, which inhibits neuronal activity. Benzodiazepines potentiate the action of GABA by binding at receptor sites of neurones. Chloride (Cl^-) ion channels in the neurone open when bound with GABA, allowing the influx of Cl^- ions from the surrounding extracellular fluid. This influx makes the neurone incapable of accepting more Cl^- ions and, as long as the channel remains open, insensitive to further stimulation. This insensitivity is what is responsible for the inhibiting effect of GABA, which is increased when BDZs are taken (Tallman et al., 2002; McGavock, 2005; Bandelow & Kaiya, 2006). All true BDZs act on GABAa receptors to exert their inhibitory effect. The main differences between them are the variations in half-lives. The length of half-lives is clinically relevant as this will influence how long the drug takes to work and for how long the effects will be apparent. It also relates to how likely a drug is to cause withdrawal effects, and its propensity for misuse as a recreational drug.

Side effects and interactions

If BDZs are not taken with other CNS depressants then they are relatively safe in overdose. If respiratory depression does occur then flumazenil can be given to reverse the effects. Flumazenil is a BDZ antagonist and should be available in clinical settings where large or injected doses of BDZs are a possibility (Carvalho & Walker, 2007; Taylor et al., 2007). The common side effects of BDZs include sedation/somnolence, headaches, confusion, ataxia (unsteadiness on feet), blurred vision, gastrointestinal problems, jaundice, amnesia and paradoxical excitement (Joint Formulary Committee, 2008). The likelihood of paradoxical excitement and behavioural disinhibition increases where someone has pre-existing tendencies for being aggressive, has a learning disability, is young or has a diagnosis of personality disorder (Taylor et al., 2007). The most serious interaction of BDZs is with other CNS depressants such as alcohol, methadone or opiates, causing a risk of respiratory depression. Benzodiazepines are metabolised by P450 liver enzymes but they do not increase or decrease the action of these enzymes and, as such, will not influence plasma levels of other drugs (Fukasawa et al., 2007). It is possible that plasma levels of BDZs can be influenced by co-administration of some other drugs (please refer to the later section on danger zones).

Caution is advised when using BDZs in the older population as older people are more susceptible to adverse effects and falls.

Tolerance and addiction

It is widely accepted that prolonged use of BDZs (over 4 weeks) is associated with physical and psychological tolerance, and addiction. The anti-anxiety and sleep-inducing properties of BDZs reduce with longer term use. As a result, greater doses of the drug are needed to exert the same effects. This is why BDZs should only be used for short periods (Joint Formulary Committee, 2008; National Institute of Clinical Excellence, 2007). The chances of addiction are reduced if the drug is used for less than 4 weeks, a BDZ with a longer half-life is used or if they are taken intermittently rather than daily.

The mechanism of action of withdrawal relates to the reduced action of GABA and the subsequent rebound stimulation of the CNS. The symptoms of withdrawal are both physical and psychological. Both groups of withdrawal symptoms can mimic some mental health problems and because of this service users may misinterpret withdrawal to be a sign of relapse. The common withdrawal symptoms include stiffness, weakness, intestinal problems, flu symptoms, visual disturbances, possible seizures, anxiety, insomnia, vivid dreams, cognitive impairment, depression and delusions/hallucinations. Benzodiazepines with shorter half-lives will induce withdrawal symptoms earlier and in a more severe form. *The Maudsley Prescribing Guidelines* (Taylor et al., 2007) provide excellent recommendations for managing BDZs withdrawal, with the initial management being to swap any shorter acting drugs to diazepam (which has a longer half-life of 20–40 h).

Other anti-anxiety medicines

Other drugs are used for the management of anxiety and any related sleep problems; the choice of drug depends on the anxiety disorder diagnosed.

The use of barbiturates to manage acute anxiety is generally avoided in clinical practice due to the possible toxic effects in overdose, which can lead to coma and death. Overdose of barbiturates can occur accidentally due the small differences between therapeutic doses and toxic doses. Barbiturates act on the same receptors to potentiate GABA as BDZs.

Buspirone is a non-benzodiazepine anxiolytic. Its mechanism of action is different to that of BDZs as it does not act on GABA receptors but exactly how it works is unclear. It appears that its therapeutic effects are related to its action on (and the relationship between) dopamine, serotonin, noradrenaline and acetylcholine. It takes around 3–6 weeks to work and therefore has no place in the acute management of anxiety. Buspirone does not appear to cause dependence and has no clinical sedative or anti-convulsant properties. Its side effects include dizziness, drowsiness, headache, insomnia, nausea, dry mouth and palpitations. Hypertensive crisis can be a consequence of taking buspirone and MAOIs, and serum levels of buspirone can be increased to toxic levels if taken with some drugs that inhibit some P450 liver enzymes (e.g. erythromycin and nefazadone).

Non-benzodiazepine hypnotics such as zopiclone and zolpidem are used to manage insomnia. However, they cause side effects similar to those of BDZs and should be used sparingly. In fact they really have no place in the treatment of anxiety disorders and are licensed only to promote sleep. Some antihistamines (e.g. promethazine) are occasionally used for their sedative properties. They work by blocking histamine H1 receptors but again they are not licensed for use in anxiety disorders.

Beta-blockers (e.g. propranalol) are sometimes used to alleviate some of the physical manifestations of anxiety. They can help to reduce tremor and palpitations but will have no direct effect on tension or sleep problems. When noradrenaline is released across a synapse it binds with a variety of receptors including beta1 and beta2. Noradrenaline acts at these receptors to increase heart rate/force and increase contraction of skeletal muscles. By blocking the action at the beta receptors the effects of noradrenaline are reduced and hence the reduction in heart rate and tremor. Non-specific beta-blockers like propranalol block beta1 and beta2 receptors, which results in constriction of the bronchioles and therefore should never be given to a service user with asthma or other respiratory problems (McGavock, 2005). Key points regarding anti-anxiety medicines can be found in Box 2.4.

Box 2.4   Anti-anxiety – key points

- The most effective treatment to promote recovery from anxiety disorders is CBT based.
- If medication is to be used it should be an SSRI in the first instance.
- Benzodiazepines are helpful to manage acute symptoms, but they are addictive and should only be used short term or on a PRN basis.
- Anxiety can be a symptom of many mental health problems; the underlying condition should be addressed to promote recovery.

Medicines for dementia

There is a wide range of drugs used to treat the variety of symptoms that can present with dementia. For example, psychotic symptoms may develop and be treated with antipsychotics although olanzapine and risperidone should not be used as they increase risk of stroke in older people with dementia (Ballard & Waite, 2006). These drugs used to treat secondary symptoms are examined elsewhere in this chapter. Dosing may be lower than normal due to lower metabolic rates in older people who make up the majority of dementia sufferers. This section examines those drugs designed to treat the cognitive impairment – largely memory deficits, which are characteristic of dementia.

Memory and learning is a highly complex function involving a multitude of pathways and a variety of neurotransmitters. As yet there is only an incomplete understanding of the processes involved. However, research has implicated the degeneration of cholinergic neurons originating in part of the amygdala called the nucleus basalis of Meynert as a major factor in the impairment of short-term memory and there seems an overall reduction in acetylcholine activity (Herholz et al., 2000; Stahl, 2000). This has led to the development of drugs designed to boost cholinergic activity to enhance cognitive function and memory impairment. These drugs are termed cholinesterase inhibitors. Three are currently licensed for use in mild –to moderate dementia in Alzheimer's disease: donepezil, galantamine and rivastigmine. One further drug, memantine, is licensed for use in moderate–to severe dementia in Alzheimer's disease but it is not a cholinesterase inhibitor.

The prescribing of these drugs has been the subject of considerable public debate. At the moment a technology appraisal by NICE recommends that they are made available in mild –to moderate Alzheimer's disease as long as certain criteria are met (see below). This has proved controversial and a legal challenge was mounted, albeit unsuccessfully, by a number of bodies including the Royal College of Nursing, the Royal College of Psychiatry, Age Concern and the Alzheimer's Society. It is of interest that a cost effectiveness study of memantine in Finland concluded that the extended independence and delay of institutionalisation amply offset the cost of treatment (Francois et al., 2004).

Mechanisms of action

Cholinesterase inhibitors inhibit the enzyme that breaks down acetylcholine called acetylcholinesterase (AChE). By doing this there is an increase in the amount of acetylcholine available. The three drugs, although achieving the same therapeutic goal, are different from one another. Donepezil is a long acting, reversible AChE inhibitor, rivastigmine is intermediate acting and pseudo-irreversible, and galantamine may have a dual action in not only inhibiting acetylcholine breakdown in a similar way, but through its agonist activity at nicotinic receptors may induce acetylcholine release (Stahl, 2000; Birks, 2006; Loy & Schneider, 2006). Memantine has a different action altogether. It is thought that a mechanism responsible for neuronal injury or death is over-exposure to the excitatory neurotransmitter glutamate. This is termed 'excitotoxicity'. One receptor involved in this process is the glutamate N-methyl-D-aspartate (NMDA) receptor. Memantine is a non-competitive, low affinity, NMDA antagonist, allowing normal activity but having the ability to regulate excess Ca^{2+} ion influx under conditions of over-activation (Lipton, 2005). This impedes the progression of symptoms.

Evidence of effectiveness

A systematic review of studies of cholinesterase inhibitors used to treat mild to moderate dementia shows that there is no notable variation between the three drugs. Small benefits were noted in activities of daily living and behaviour as well as assessment scales. Similar benefits were also noted in cases of severe dementia but the number of studies (two) is too small to draw conclusions (Birks et al., 2000; Birks, 2006; Loy & Schneider, 2006). However small the benefits may appear, it can be argued that small or indeed no benefits over a period of 6 months, the timescale of a number of trials, constitutes a therapeutic success in what is a progressively degenerative disease.

Side effects

The most common side effects of cholinesterase inhibitors are gastrointestinal. These include nausea, vomiting and diarrhoea. Others such as headaches, insomnia, dizziness and psychiatric disturbances may also occur. Memantine can cause constipation, headaches, drowsiness and dizziness. Less commonly it can induce vomiting, confusion, hallucinations and fatigue. Seizures have also been reported but very rarely.

Interactions

The drugs for dementia have few strong interactions. Memantine has an increased risk of causing CNS toxicity when given with amantadine, ketamine or dextromethorphan and it is recommended that they are not used together. Galantamine may have its plasma concentration levels increased by a number of drugs, notably paroxetine and erythromycin. Key points regarding dementia and Alzheimer's disease can be found in Boxes 2.5 and 2.6, respectively.

Box 2.5   Dementia – key points

- Prescribing should concur with the relevant guidance.
- Co-morbidity is common in older people and care should be taken with possible interactions.
- Lower metabolic rates may affect dosing regimes.

Box 2.6   NICE guidance

The three drugs donepezil, rivastigmine and galantamine should be made available in the NHS as one component of the management of those people with mild and moderate Alzheimer's disease (AD) whose mini mental state examination (MMSE) score is above 10 points under the following conditions:

- Diagnosis that the form of dementia is AD must be made in a specialist clinic according to standard diagnostic criteria.
- Assessment in a specialist clinic, including tests of cognitive, global and behavioural functioning and of activities of daily living, should be made before the drug is prescribed.
- Clinicians should also exercise judgement about the likelihood of compliance; in general, a carer or care-worker that is in sufficient contact with the patient to ensure compliance should be a minimum requirement.
- Only specialists (including old-age psychiatrists, neurologists and care of older people physicians) should initiate treatment. Carers' views of the patient's condition at baseline and follow-up should be sought. If general practitioners are to take over prescribing, it is recommended that they should do so under an agreed shared-care protocol with clear treatment end points.
- A further assessment should be made, usually 2 to 4 months after reaching maintenance dose of the drug. Following this assessment the drug should be continued only where there has been an improvement or no deterioration in MMSE score, together with evidence of global improvement on the basis of behavioural and/or functional assessment.
- Patients who continue on the drug should be reviewed by MMSE score and global, functional and behavioural assessment every 6 months. The drug should normally only be continued while their MMSE score remains above 10 points, and their global, functional and behavioural condition remains at a level where the drug is considered to be having a worthwhile effect. When the MMSE score falls below 10 points, patients should not normally be prescribed any of these three drugs. Any review involving MMSE assessment should be undertaken by an appropriate specialist team, unless there are locally agreed protocols for shared care.
- The benefits of these three drugs for patients with other forms of dementia (e.g. Dementia with Lewy Bodies) was not assessed in the guidance.

Adapted from NICE – NICE technology appraisal guidance 111 (amended), 2007.

Danger zones – areas of risk with psychotropics

As previously discussed, all psychotropics can cause unwanted effects and can interact with other medications. Side effects are distressing to service users and influence adherence with treatment; however, some undesired effects are potentially fatal and warrant further exploration. Some of the serious reactions to medications are predictable and, if identified early, can be managed to reduce the risk of serious harm occurring.

Drug interactions are generally pharmacodynamic or pharmacokinetic in nature and can occur with psychotropic and other medications. Pharmacodynamic interactions are when two drugs act at the same neurotransmitter site or the same organ. For example, MAOIs with SSRIs both increase serotonin and can cause serotonin syndrome. Similarly, using TCAs and some antipsychotics together may cause an increased risk of cardiac arrhythmias. Pharmacokinetic interactions are where two drugs influence the way the drugs are absorbed, distributed, metabolised or eliminated in the body. For simplicity we have focused on the main psychotropic drugs, but if a service user is prescribed a combination of drugs, possible interactions should always be checked.

P450 liver enzyme interactions

We have already briefly mentioned some of the potential interactions due to changes in metabolism because of the way drugs influence P450 liver enzymes. If the mechanism of these interactions is understood and interactions between co-prescribed drugs are checked many of these problems can be avoided. There are a variety of cytochrome P450 liver enzymes that are either solely or sometimes jointly responsible for the metabolism of fat-soluble medicines in the body. Some drugs induce P450 enzymes, which results in reduced serum levels of drugs that are also metabolised by the same enzyme. Because of this a P450 inducer can result in sub-therapeutic blood levels and possible treatment failure. Other drugs inhibit P450, which results in higher blood levels of drugs metabolised by the same P450 enzyme, leading to possible dangerously toxic levels of drugs. Genetic differences can also influence the action of P450 liver enzymes and this can lead to the same complications as drug-induced interactions (McGavock, 2005).

Lithium toxicity

Lithium toxicity occurs when the level of lithium in the blood becomes too high. The effects occur at blood levels in excess of 1.5 mmol/l and are potentially fatal. The desired serum level for therapeutic effects is around 0.4–1.0 mmol/l. As previously discussed, lithium blood levels should be monitored 3–6 monthly when the desired serum level is achieved.

The signs of lithium toxicity include shaking and trembling, confusion, slurred speech, nausea and vomiting, diarrhoea, abdominal pain, unsteadiness on the feet, coma, seizures and possible death. People who have lithium toxicity usually look sick, pale, grey and weak (Taylor et al., 2007). If toxicity is suspected, immediately refer/accompany the service user for a check of serum levels (accident and emergency (A&E) if regular services are unavailable), advise them to drink water and not take the medicine until seen by a doctor.

Increased levels of lithium can occur in service users that are at a steady blood level. The common causes include any dehydration, low levels of dietary salt and interactions with other drugs (diuretics, NSAIDs, SSRIs, carbamazepine and ACE inhibitors).

Advising and sharing information with service users can help prevent toxicity. The following points should be made clear:

- Have regular blood tests.
- Drink plenty of fluids – at least six glasses of water daily.
- Drink extra water in cases of hot weather, strenuous exercise or vomiting/diarrhoea.
- Do not start a salt-reduced diet whilst taking lithium.
- Do not take double doses if a dose is forgotten.
- Do not take over-the-counter or herbal medicines without first consulting a health professional.
- Be alert to the signs of toxicity and contact key-worker or go to A&E if concerned.

QTc interval issues

Many medicines have an effect on cardiac functioning. Psychotropic drugs in particular are associated with prolongation of the QTc interval, which may induce arrhythmias and can lead to a condition called Torsades de pointes (TDP) or 'twisted points,' a graphic description of the ECG trace appearance (Calderone et al., 2005). This in turn may lead to sudden death (Hippius, 1999; Stollberger et al., 2005). QTc prolongation is caused by the blocking of the HERG *I* kr potassium channel. A wide variety of antipsychotics have been shown to cause this, as well as other types of drugs such as tricyclic antidepressants. Group 2 phenothiazines, particularly thioridazine, and high doses generally (Warner et al., 1996) are prone to inducing this problem and it has been a cause of concern for a number of atypical antipsychotics such as sertindole.

Blood dyscrasias

Virtually all psychotropic medications have been associated with haematological adverse effects. Although blood-related side effects are relatively rare they have the potential to be fatal. These adverse effects are most likely to occur early on in treatment. Agranulocytosis, for example, usually happens 21–28 days after starting psychotropics (Oyesanmi et al., 1999).

A variety of blood-related adverse effects can be caused by psychotropic medications. The exact mechanisms behind these effects are still debated but may relate to bone marrow suppression, toxicity of the bone marrow directly relating to the drug and the destruction of immune cells. The blood dyscrasias most commonly associated with psychotropic medication include agranulocytosis (bone marrow no longer produces leucocytes), neutropenia (low neutrophil count), aplastic anaemia (insufficient blood cells for circulation) and minimal changes in red blood cell counts. All these disorders can result in an inability to fight infection and can leave the individual at risk of acquiring opportunistic infections. When managing any psychotropic medication clinicians need to be particularly alert for signs of infection. A full blood count should be conducted periodically and at the first signs of infection.

Clozapine is perhaps the most well-known drug to cause haematological adverse effects (and as a result it is associated with regular monitoring), but almost all classes of antipsychotics can cause blood-related adverse effects. Of the first generation antipsychotics, chlorpromazine, fluphenazine, haloperidol and loxapine have all been associated with a variety of blood disorders. Clozapine, olanzapine and risperidone are second-generation antipsychotics that have been reported to cause blood dyscrasias (other antipsychotic agents may also cause similar problems but as clinical experience with these is limited, the exact risk remains to be seen). Recent risk estimates suggest that clozapine causes agranulocytosis in 0.8% of cases and chlorpromazine in around 0.13% of cases (Flanagan & Dunk, 2008).

Antidepressants can also cause an array of blood-related side effects. Agranulocytosis has been reported with tricyclic antidepressants (mainly imipramine) although this is with less frequency than with antipsychotris (Oyensanmi et al., 1999). Clinicians should be especially aware that the initial symptoms of agranulocytosis can look similar to depression and as a result may be misidentified as being mood related. SSRI antidepressants have been associated with increased bruising and bleeding relating to impaired platelet aggregation, and rarely with agranulocytosis. The overall incidence of depleted white blood cells associated with antidepressants has been estimated at 0.01% (Stubner et al., 2004).

The risk of developing blood-related adverse effects with anti-convulsants is higher than with antidepressants. Carbamazepine can cause initial transient reductions in white cells in around 10% of cases and this progresses to cause neutropenia in 0.5% of cases; as a result carbamazepine and clozapine should not be prescribed concurrently (Flanagan & Dunk, 2008).

Due to the real possibility of service users developing blood-related disorders associated with psychotropics, all clinicians should be alert to the relevant signs and symptoms and ensure that routine blood monitoring is carried out. Stopping the psychotropic associated with blood dyscrasias will usually result in a resolution of symptoms, although all cases should be assessed and treated by a specialist as required.

Conclusion

It is clear that the pharmacology of drugs used across the spectrum of mental illness is complex. Despite continuing to attract controversy, there is no doubt that symptoms can be alleviated and distress reduced for many people through the appropriate use of psychotropic medication. However, it is also clear that there is a wide range of problems associated with their use. Understanding the pharmacology of the drugs we use is an essential part of our professional role which enables us to act as a resource for our clients, promoting informed decisions, maximising the therapeutic potential and minimising any negative impact of the treatment for their benefit.

References

Ananth, J., Parameswaran, S. & Gunatilake, S. (2004) Side effects of atypical antipsychotic drugs. *Current Pharmaceutical Design*, **10**(18), 2219–2229.

Ashton, A.K., Jamerson, B.D., Weinstein, W.L. & Wagoner, C. (2005) Antidepressant-related adverse effects impacting treatment compliance: results of a patient survey. *Current Therapeutic Research*, **66**(2), 96–106.

Ballard, C. & Waite, J. (2006) The effectiveness of atypical antipsychotics for the treatment of aggression and psychosis in Alzheimer's disease. In: *Cochrane Database of Systematic Reviews*. John Wiley & Sons, Ltd., Chichester.

Bandelow, B. & Kaiya, H. (2006) Drug treatment for panic disorder. *International Congress Series*, **1287**, 288–292.

Baylis, P.H. & Heath, D.A. (1978) Water disturbances in patients treated with oral lithium carbonate. *Annals of Internal Medicine*, **88**(5), 607–609.

Birks, J. (2006) Cholinesterase inhibitors for Alzheimer's disease. In: *Cochrane Database of Systematic Reviews*. John Wiley & Sons Ltd, Chichester.

Birks, J., Grimley, E.J., Lakovidou, V. & Tsolaki, M. (2000) Rivastigmine for Alzheimer's disease. In: *Cochrane Database of Systematic Reviews*. John Wiley & Sons Ltd, Chichester.

Brill, M. (2004) Antidepressants and sexual dysfunction. *Sexuality, Reproduction & Menopause*, **2**(1), 35–40.

Burgess, S., Geddes, J., Hawton, K., Townsend, E., Jamison, K. & Goodwin, G. (2001) Lithium for maintenance treatment of mood disorders. In: *Cochrane Database of Systematic Reviews*. John Wiley & Sons Ltd, Chichester.

Calderone, V., Testai, L., Martinotti, E., Del Tacca, M. & Breschi, M.C. (2005) Drug induced block of cardiac HERG potassium channels and development of torsade de pointes arrythmias; the case for antipsychotics. *Journal of Pharmacy and Pharmacology*, **57**(2), 151–161.

Caroff, S.N. & Mann, S.C. (1993) Neuroleptic malignant syndrome. *The Medical Clinics of North America*, **77**(1), 185–202.

Carvalho, C. & Walker, D. (2007) Coma cocktail; a role for flumazenil. *British Journal of Hospital Medicine*, **68**(2), 112.

Chengappa, K.N., Suppes, T. & Berk, M. (2004) Treatment of bipolar mania with atypical antipsychotics. *Expert Review of Neurotherapeutics*, **4**(no. 6 Suppl 2), S17–S25.

Cipriani, A., Pretty, H., Hawton, K. & Geddes, J.R. (2005) Lithium in the prevention of suicidal behavior and all-cause mortality in patients with mood disorders: a systematic review of randomized trials. *American Journal of Psychiatry*, **162**(10), 1805–1819.

Cunningham-Owens, D.G. (1999) *A Guide to the Extrapyramidal Side Effects of Antipsychotic Drugs*. Cambridge University Press, Cambridge.

Davies, M.A., Sheffler, D.J. & Roth, B.L. (2004) Aripiprazole: a novel atypical antipsychotic drug with a uniquely robust pharmacology. *CNS Drug Reviews*, **10**(4), 317–336.

De Soto, M.F., Griffith, S.R. & Katz, E.J. (1985) Water intoxication associated with nephrogenic diabetes insipidus secondary to lithium: case report. *Journal of Clinical Psychiatry*, **46**(9), 402–403.

Desarkar, P., Thakur, A. & Sinha, V.K. (2006) Aripiprazole-induced acute dystonia. *American Journal of Psychiatry*, **163**(6), 1112–1113.

El-Sayeh, H.G. & Morganti, C. (2006) Aripiprazole for schizophrenia. In: *Cochrane Database of Systematic Reviews*. John Wiley & Sons Ltd, Chichester.

Eustatia-Rutten, C.F., Tamsma, J.T. & Meinders, A.E. (2001) Lithium-induced nephrogenic diabetes insipidus. *Netherlands Journal of Medicine*, **58**(3), 137–142.

Flanagan, R.J. & Dunk, L. (2008) Haematological toxicity of drugs used in psychiatry. *Human Psychopharmacology*, **23**(Suppl 1), 27–41.

Fleischhacker, W.W. (2005) Aripiprazole. *Expert Opinion on Pharmacotherapy*, **6**(12), 2091–2101.

Francois, C., Sintonen, H., Sulkava, R. & Rive, B. (2004) Cost effectiveness of memantine in moderately severe to severe Alzheimer's disease: A Markov model in Finland. *Clinical Drug Investigation*, **24**(7), 373–384.

Fukasawa, T., Suzuki, A. & Otani, K. (2007) Effects of genetic polymorphism of cytochrome P450 enzymes on the pharmacokinetics of benzodiazepines. *Journal of Clinical Pharmacy and Therapeutics*, **32**(4), 333–341.

Gardner, D.M., Baldessarini, R.J. & Waraich, P. (2005) Modern antipsychotic drugs: a critical overview. *Canadian Medical Association Journal*, **172**(13), 1703–1711.

Geddes, J., Freemantle, N., Harrison, P. & Bebbington, P. (2000) Atypical antipsychotics in the treatment of schizophrenia: systematic overview and meta-regression analysis. *British Medical Journal*, **321**, 1371–1376.

Ghaemi, S.N., Hsu, D.J., Rosenquist, K.J., Pardo, T.B. & Goodwin, F.K. (2006) Extrapyramidal side-effect effects with atypical neuroleptics in bipolar disorder. *Progress in Neuro-Psychopharmacology & Biological Psychiatry*, **30**(2), 209–213.

Gilman, P.K. (2006) A review of serotonin toxicity data: implications for the mechanisms of antidepressant drug action. *Journal of Biological Psychiatry*, **59,** 1046–1051.

Goodwin, G.M. & Geddes, J.R. (2003) Latest maintenance data on lithium in bipolar disorder. *European Neuropsychopharmacology*, **13**(Suppl 2), 51–55.

Gurvich, N. & Klein, P.S. (2002) Lithium and valproic acid: parallels and contrasts in diverse signaling contexts. *Pharmacology & Therapeutics*, **96**(1), 45–66.

Haddad, P.M. & Anderson, I.M. (2007) Recognising and managing antidepressant discontinuation symptoms. *Advances in Psychiatric Treatment*, **13**, 447–457.

Herholz, K., Bauer, B., Wienhard, K., et al. (2000) In-vivo measurements of regional acetylcholine esterase activity in degenerative dementia: comparison with blood flow and glucose metabolism. *Journal of Neural Transmission*, **107**(12), 1457–1468.

Hermesh, H., Aizenberg, D., Weizman, A., Lapidot, M., Mayor, C. & Munitz, H. (1992) Risk for definite neuroleptic malignant syndrome. A prospective study in 223 consecutive in-patients. *British Journal of Psychiatry*, **161**, 254–257.

Hippius, H. (1999) A historical perspective of clozapine. *Journal of Clinical Psychiatry*, **60**(Suppl 12), 22–23.

Hirose, T. & Kikuchi, T. (2005) Aripiprazole, a novel antipsychotic agent: dopamine D2 receptor partial agonist. *Journal of Medical Investigation*, **52**(Suppl 90), 284–290.

Holmes, D.S. (1994) *Abnormal Psychology.* Harper Collins, New York.

Illowsky, B.P. & Kirch, D.G. (1988) Polydipsia and hyponatremia in psychiatric patients. *American Journal of Psychiatry*, **145**(6), 675–683.

Joint Formulary Committee (2008) *British National Formulary.* British Medical Association and Royal Pharmaceutical Society of Great Britain, London.

Kennedy, S.H., Dickens, S.E., Eisfeld, B.S. & Bagby, R.M. (1999) Sexual dysfunction before antidepressant therapy in major depression. *Journal of Affective Disorders*, **56**, 201–208.

Kikkert, M.J,. Schene, A.H., Koeter, M.W.J., et al. (2006) Medication adherence in schizophrenia: exploring patients', carers' and professionals' views. *Schizophrenia Bulletin*, **32**(4), 786–794.

Kleindienst, N. & Greil, W. (2003) Lithium in the long-term treatment of bipolar disorders. *European Archives of Psychiatry & Clinical Neuroscience*, **253**(3), 120–125.

Kontaxakis, V.P., Ferentinos, P.P., Havaki-Kontaxaki, B.J. & Roukas, D.K. (2005) Randomized controlled augmentation trials in clozapine-resistant schizophrenic patients: a critical review. *European Psychiatry*, **20**(5–6), 409–415.

Kosten, T.R. & Forrest, J.N. (1986) Treatment of severe lithium-induced polyuria with amiloride. *American Journal of Psychiatry*, **143**(12), 1563–1568.

Lejoyeux, M., Rouillon, F. & Ades, J. (1993) Prospective evaluation of the serotonin syndrome in depressed inpatients treated with clomipramine. *Acta Psychiatrica Scandinavica*, **88**, 369–371.

Lenox, R.H. & Wang, L. (2003) Molecular basis of lithium action: integration of lithium-responsive signaling and gene expression networks. *Molecular Psychiatry*, **8**, 135–144.

Leonard, B. & Richelson, E. (2003) Synaptic effects of antidepressants: relation to their therapeutic and adverse effects. In Buckley, P.F. & Waddington, J.L. (eds) *In Schizophrenia and Mood Disorders: The New Drug Therapies in Clinical Practice*. Butterworth-Heinemann, Oxford.

Linde, K., Mulrow, C.D., Berner, M. & Egger, M. (2005) St John's Wort for depression. In: *Cochrane Database of Systematic Reviews*. John Wiley & Sons Ltd, Chichester.

Lipton, S.A. (2005) The molecular basis of memantine action in Alzheimer's disease and other neurologic disorders: low-affinity, uncompetitive antagonism. *Current Alzheimer Research*, **2**(2), 155–165.

Loy, C. & Schneider, L. (2006) Galantamine for Alzheimer's disease and mild cognitive impairment. In: *Cochrane Database of Systematic Reviews*. John Wiley & Sons Ltd, Chichester.

Macritchie, K., Geddes, J.R., Scott, J., Haslam, D., de Lima, M. & Goodwin, G. (2003) Valproate for acute mood episodes in bipolar disorder. In: *Cochrane Database of Systematic Reviews*. John Wiley & Sons Ltd, Chichester.

Macritchie, K.A., Geddes, J.R., Scott, J., Haslam, D.R. & Goodwin, G.M. (2001) Valproic acid, valproate and divalproex in the maintenance treatment of bipolar disorder. In: *Cochrane Database of Systematic Reviews*. John Wiley & Sons Ltd, Chichester.

Margolese, H.C., Chouinard, G., Kolivakis, T.T., Beauclair, L., Miller, R. & Annable, L. (2005) Tardive dyskinesia in the era of typical and atypical antipsychotics. Part 2: Incidence and management strategies in patients with schizophrenia. *Canadian Journal of Psychiatry*, **50**(11), 703–714.

Marken, P.A. & Pies, R.W. (2006) Emerging treatments for bipolar disorder: safety and adverse effect profiles. *Annals of Pharmacotherapy*, **40**(2), 276–285.

McGahuey, A.J., Gelenberg, C.A., Lankes, F.A., Moreno & Delgado, P.L. (2000) The Arizona Sexual Experiences Scale (ASEX) Reliability and validity. *Journal of Sex & Marital Therapy*, **26**(1), 25–40.

McGarry, H., Pirotta, M., Hegarty, K. & Gunn, J. (2006) General practitioners and St. John's Wort: A question of regulation or knowledge? *Complementary Therapies in Medicine*, **15**(2), 142–148.

McGavock, H. (2005) *How Drugs Work – Basic Pharmacology for Health Care Professionals*. Radcliffe Publishing, Oxford.

McKay, A.P. & McKenna, P.J. (1993) The dopamine hypothesis of schizophrenia. *Clinician*, **11**(4), 31–42.

Mendhekar, D.N. (2005) Ziprasidone-induced tardive dyskinesia. *Canadian Journal of Psychiatry*, **50**(9), 567–568.

Mennin, T. & Gobbi, M. (2004) The antidepressant mechanism of *Hypericum perforatum*. *Life Sciences*, **75**(9), 1021–1027.

Mir, S. & Taylor, D. (2001) Atypical antipsychotics and hyperglycaemia. *International Clinical Psychopharmacology*, **16**(2), 63–73.

National Collaborating Centre for Mental Health. (2003) *Schizophrenia: Full National Clinical Guideline on Core Interventions in Primary and Secondary Care*. Royal College of Psychiatrists and The British Psychological Society, London.

National Institute for Health and Clinical Excellence. (2004) *Anxiety (amended) Management of anxiety (panic disorder with or without agoraphobia and GAD) in adults*. NICE clinical guideline 22, London.

National Institute of Clinical Excellence. (2002) *Guidance on the use of newer (atypical) antipsychotic drugs for the treatment of schizophrenia*. NICE, London.

National Institute of Clinical Excellence (2004) *Depression: Management of depression in primary and secondary care. Clinical guideline 23*. NICE, London.

National Institute of Clinical Excellence (2007) *Donepezil, galantamine, rivastigmine (review) and memantine for the treatment of Alzheimer's disease (amended), includes a review of NICE technology appraisal guidance 19*. NICE technology appraisal guidance 111 (amended). NICE, London.

Nguyen, L.N. & Guthrie, S.K. (2006) Risperidone treatment of bipolar mania. *Annals of Pharmacotherapy*, **40**(4), 674–682.

Oyesanmi, O., Kunkel, E.J.S., Monti, D.A. & Field, H.L. (1999) Hematologic side effects of psychotropics. *Psychosomatics*, **40**, 414–421.

Pini, S., Abelli, M. & Cassano, G.B. (2006) The role of quetiapine in the treatment of bipolar disorder. *Expert Opinion on Pharmacotherapy*, **7**(7), 929–940.

Remington, G., Saha, A., Chong, S.A. & Shammi, C. (2005) Augmentation strategies in clozapine-resistant schizophrenia. *CNS Drugs*, **19**(10), 843–872.

Sanders, R.D. & Mossman, D. (1999) An open trial of olanzapine in patients with treatment-refractory psychoses. *Journal of Clinical Psychopharmacology*, **19**(1), 62–66.

Sharma, A. & Sorrell, J.H. (2006) Aripiprazole-induced parkinsonism. *International Clinical Psychopharmacology*, **21**(2), 127–129.

Simon, G.E. (2002) Evidence review: efficacy and effectiveness of antidepressant treatment in primary care. *General Hospital Psychiatry*, **24**(4), 213–224.

Stahl, S. (2000) *Essential Psychopharmacology. Neuroscientific Basis and Practical Applications*. Cambridge University Press, Cambridge.

Stollberger, C., Huber, J.O. & Finsterer, J. (2005) Antipsychotic drugs and QT prolongation. *International Clinical Psychopharmacology*, **20**(5), 243–251.

Stubner, S., Grohmann, R., Engel, R., et al. (2004) Blood dyscrasias induced by psychotropic drugs. *Pharmacopsychiatry*, **37**(Suppl 1), 70–78.

Tallman, J., Cassella, J. & Kehne, J. (2002) Mechanism of action of anxiolytics. In Davis, K., Charney, D., Coyle, J. & Nameroff, C. (eds) *Neuropsychopharmacology: The Fifth Generation of Progress*. Lippincott, Williams & Wilkins, Philadelphia.

Taylor, D., Paton, C. & Kerwin, R. (2007) *The Maudsley Prescribing Guidelines 2006–200* Taylor and Francis group, London.

Vaswani, M., Farzana, K.L. & Subramanyam Ramesh, R. (2003) Role of selective serotonin reuptake inhibitors in psychiatric disorders: a comprehensive review. *Progress in Neuro-Psychopharmacology & Biological Psychiatry*, **27**, 85–102.

Verhoeven, W.M.A., Doesburg, W.H., Snoej, R., Rutgers, A.J.M.P. & Van Dongen, P.H.M. (1992) Efficacy of clozapine in treatment-resistant psychosis and neuroleptic sensitivity: Results of the Dutch open multi-center project. *European Psychiatry*, **7**(2), 77–84.

Vieta, E. & Goikolea, J.M. (2005) Atypical antipsychotics: newer options for mania and maintenance therapy. *Bipolar Disorders*, **7**(Suppl 4), 21–33.

Wahlbeck, K., Cheine, M.V. & Essali, A. (1999) Clozapine versus typical neuroleptic medication for schizophrenia. In: *Cochrane Database of Systematic Reviews*. John Wiley & Sons Ltd, Chichester.

Warner, J.P., Barnes, T.R. & Henry, J.A. (1996) Electrocardiographic changes in patients receiving neuroleptic medication. *Acta Psychiatrica Scandinavica*, **93**, 311–313.

Wolf, R., Tscherne, U. & Emrich, H.M. (1988) Suppression of preoptic GABA release caused by push-pull-perfusion with sodium valproate. *Naunyn-Schmiedebergs Archives of Pharmacology*, **338**(6), 658–663.

Zacher, J.L. & Hatchett, A.D. (2006) Aripiprazole-induced movement disorder. *American Journal of Psychiatry*, **163**(1), 160–161.

Ziegenbein, M., Sieberer, M., Calliess, I.T. & Kropp, S. (2006) Aripiprazole-induced extrapyramidal side-effect effects in a patient with schizoaffective disorder. *Australian & New Zealand Journal of Psychiatry*, **40**(2), 194–195.

3

Drug interactions and co-morbidity

Jenny Blackshaw and Petra Brown

Introduction

The fact that many drugs interact with each other is well known. Considerable time and expense have been invested in researching potential interactions between medicines and conditions, both during the development of new pharmacological treatments and once marketed. The pharmacological basis for many drug interactions is also well known. Interactions can be anticipated in many cases through knowing the action of drugs in the body and brain. However, these expected interactions sometimes do not occur clinically and, conversely, there are times when interactions and adverse effects occur without warning (Royal College of Psychiatrists, 2005). Interactions can also occur with non-prescribed drugs (substances). There is potential for interactions between prescribed and illicit substances, smoking and alcohol. Examples and case reports are documented in various texts and literature. From knowing the mode of action of many of these substances, it is possible to extrapolate this information and draw conclusions about possible effects and adverse effects that will occur when they are taken concurrently.

Unfortunately, research in this area is scarce. The reasons for this are multi-factorial: firstly, medicines research is expensive and often sponsored by the pharmaceutical industry; secondly, medicines research is conducted in compliant persons and excludes many groups, especially those with substance misuse or alcohol problems; finally, there is considerable difficulty in getting accurate and truthful histories of what substances have been taken. Aside from these considerations other factors need to be considered, including: how many different substances have been taken and what effect these may have had on each other, other co-morbid and physical health conditions, and variables such as age, sex and ethnicity which are known to affect the way the body handles medicines.

Drug interactions

An interaction is said to occur when the effect of one drug is changed by the presence of another:

> *'Two or more drugs given at the same time may exert their effects independently or may interact. The interaction may be potentiation or antagonism of one drug by another, or occasionally some other "effect"'*

Joint Formulary Committee (2008)

Drug interactions can essentially work in three ways: they can make a drug less effective, cause unexpected side effects or increase the effect of a certain drug.

There are numerous examples of these three mechanisms; the following hope to explain the concept. Further examples more specific to working with a service user with a dual diagnosis can be found later in this chapter.

Two drugs making each less effective

Amphetamines and antipsychotics have been known to negate the effects of each other. This could be postulated from the known pharmacological effect on dopamine receptors but has also been seen clinically. The challenge for all clinicians is what advice should be given to a service user with, for example, schizophrenia. The use of amphetamines increases dopamine levels, which in turn can lead to a relapse or psychotic episode. All antipsychotics have an effect on dopamine to reduce levels circulating in the brain. It is assumed that this reduction in dopamine alleviates the symptoms experienced by the service user; however, it will also reduce the 'high' experienced with the amphetamine. Many reduce or discontinue their antipsychotic medication to manage this interaction. Each drug makes the other less effective.

Unexpected side effects

On occasion a side effect or adverse effect occurs unexpectedly. An example here could be the documented unexpected reaction to benzodiazepines where a usually calm person becomes aggressive, hostile or agitated. This would not be the expected effect of benzodiazepines and would not be predicted from their mode of action.

Increase the effect of a certain drug

This is seen frequently, for example when two different drugs both have a sedative side effect (such as alcohol and benzodiazepines) or drugs which both cause respiratory depression – alcohol and opiates.

Considerations for potential interactions

Even when interactions are known to be likely to occur, at times a risk assessment can suggest that the condition being treated can become more serious if left untreated than the risk posed by the possible interaction. The following are questions that should be considered by any clinician, whether prescribing, dispensing or administering medicines with regards to potential interactions (Box 3.1).

Once the points in Box 3.1 have been considered and a risk assessment undertaken, an explanation of the risks and benefits should be fully provided to the service user. This explanation should include all prescribed, purchased or illicit substances as well as nicotine and alcohol.

Box 3.1   Considerations for potential interactions

- Do we know about all the preparations the person is taking?
- Are the drugs known to interact?
- If they do, how serious is it?
- Has it been described only once or many times?
- Are all patients affected or only a few?
- What alternative/safer drugs can be used instead?
- The more medicines a patient takes the greater the chance of an adverse drug reaction.
- The incidence of problems is higher in older people and those with co-morbid conditions.

Three main types of interactions

Interactions between prescribed drugs occur in three main ways:

- *Drug/drug interactions.* These occur when two or more drugs react with each other when taken concomitantly. Examples include fluvoxamine antidepressant (selective serotonin re-uptake inhibitor,

SSRI) and clozapine (an atypical antipsychotic). When fluvoxamine is started in a service user prescribed and taking clozapine, serum levels of clozapine may increase.

- *Drug/food/drink.* Some prescribed medicines can interact with alcohol or certain foods or drinks. In addition to the direct sedating effect of alcohol, the effect of alcohol on the liver can reduce the enzymes in the liver and therefore the body's ability to break down medicines for excretion from the body. This can cause medicines that would normally be broken down in the liver to build up to possibly toxic levels. Other drugs are known to interact with cranberry or grapefruit juice, for example clozapine, clomipramine and diazepam (Bazire, 2007).
- *Drug/condition interactions.* This is where a certain medical condition can make some drugs more harmful. Epilepsy is an example where drugs known to lower the seizure threshold can cause a service user with well-maintained epilepsy to have a seizure. The tricyclic antidepressants (amitriptyline) are known to increase seizure risk in epilepsy.

Two categories of drug interactions

The above types of interactions can also be categorised into pharmacodynamic and pharmacokinetic.

- Pharmacodynamic is where the pharmacological effects of one drug are changed by the presence of another, e.g. sedation or constipation.
- Pharmacokinetic is where the processes by which drugs are absorbed, distributed, metabolised or excreted are affected by the presence of another drug, substance or condition.

Pharmacodynamic drug interaction – an example

The tricyclic antidepressant amitriptyline affects a range of systems. Because of this, interactions with other drugs and conditions can occur frequently. If amitriptyline is co-prescribed with the following, interactions and potentiation of effects can easily occur.

Amitriptyline is known to:

- block histamine H1 receptors (as does chlorphenamine) – added drowsiness;
- lower seizure threshold (as does clozapine) – seizures possible;
- affect heart rhythm (as does haloperidol) – arrhythmias.

Pharmacokinetic drug interactions – some examples

1. Some medicines are produced to dissolve in a certain part of the gastrointestinal tract. Changes to the pH (acidity) in the stomach, or changes to the speed medicines pass through the gastrointestinal tract, can affect the ability of the body to break down and then absorb them into the bloodstream.
2. Substances are distributed through the bloodstream on proteins, which carry the medicines/substances around the bloodstream to the required site of action. These can be affected by other drugs or substances that preferentially bind to the proteins in the blood, displacing the original substance. Therefore, any changes in this process will limit the amount of active medicine available.
3. Metabolism is the way a drug is broken down in the liver. Changing the amount or activity of liver enzymes is the most common cause of interactions between drugs. This is considered in greater detail later in this chapter.
4. Drugs are often excreted through the kidneys, and can be adversely affected by medicines/drugs that affect the way the body eliminates substances from the body.

Most drugs are broken down to inactive compounds by the liver. However, some medicines, such as lithium, are excreted more or less unchanged by the kidneys. Therefore, any effects on kidney function can lead to changes in excretion of these drugs and build-up of levels in the body. Becoming dehydrated when on lithium can lead to lithium toxicity, as lithium is not removed from the body as readily as usual. This has been seen at 'raves' when substances such as ecstasy have been taken. A combination of dancing, overheating, not drinking enough and lithium has led to lithium toxicity.

Cytochrome P450 and metabolism in the liver

The liver is the site where drugs are metabolised. There are 36+ isoenzymes of cytochrome P450 and four of these are responsible for breaking down over 90% of common medicines. The isoenzymes are responsible for breaking the drugs down into metabolites (break-down products) of the original drug, which allows them to be removed from the body. Effects on the liver enzymes can lead to many changes in drugs levels and interactions. The medicine/illicit substances to be broken down by the P450 system in the liver are known as the substrate. A certain isoenzyme will be responsible for the metabolism. The presence at this point of a second substance/medicine can affect the way the isoenzyme acts upon the substrate. The second substrate can either:

- speed up (enhance) the activity or quantity of the isoenzyme, therefore leading it to work more efficiently, breaking down the substrate more quickly and leaving less in the body; or
- slow down (inhibit) the activity or quantity of the isoenzyme, therefore leading to a loss of efficacy and a decrease in the rate of breakdown of the substrate. This leads to higher levels in the body.

Either of the above interactions can be dangerous, causing the service user to have either sub-therapeutic or toxic levels of a medicine in the body.

Smoking and interactions

With the advent of smoke-free spaces, support and encouragement to stop smoking has never been higher. Smoking tobacco, in cigarettes or as the vehicle for the consumption of cannabis, has a significant effect on the liver enzymes, and therefore changes in smoking habits can have a significant effect on therapeutic drug levels. Smoking a cigarette leads to the body being exposed to carbon monoxide, carbon dioxide, nicotine and polycyclic aromatic hydrocarbons. Polycylic hydrocarbons are a collection of hundreds of different chemicals that are toxic to the body. They are metabolised in the liver by the P450 system. The more cigarettes smoked the more polycyclic hydrocarbons the liver is required to metabolise. The liver increases the amount of isoenzymes to deal with this high level of polycyclic hydrocarbons. In turn, this higher level of isoenzymes affects drug metabolism.

The majority of psychotropic agents prescribed in mental health are broken down to some extent by these isoenzymes. Therefore, if a service user smokes heavily, the level of enzymes in the liver is higher, which causes the psychotropic drugs prescribed to be broken down more rapidly. This means less drug is available in the body and can lead to sub-therapeutic levels of medication.

The converse occurs when quitting smoking. Levels of polycyclic hydrocarbons decrease, leading to a reduction in the amount of liver enzymes breaking down the psychotropic agent and a subsequent increase in plasma levels of the medicine. This can lead to toxicity and/or adverse effects as metabolism returns to predicted levels. Nicotine replacement therapy (NRT) stops the physical withdrawal experienced when stopping smoking due to the addiction to nicotine. Nicotine replacement therapy does not protect from any effects on liver enzymes and therefore NRT will not protect the service user from possible changes in drug levels. Although many drugs are affected by stopping smoking, the significance varies greatly depending on the drug in question.

The timescale in which these changes occur is also significant. On stopping smoking it will take approximately 7 days before levels of liver enzymes stabilise, with any subsequent rise in drug levels taking up to a further 7 days. Practical advice therefore needs to be given to anyone quitting smoking regarding possible adverse effects to medication or recurrence of previous adverse effects. These would take a fortnight before they occurred with many medicines.

Further information on potential interactions is contained in Table 3.1.

The extent of the problem

To help put into context the issue of mental health and substance use that leads to interactions, it is worth noting the following figures:

- 26% of the general adult population drink above safe drinking levels (point prevalence);
- 27% use illicit drugs (lifetime prevalence);
- 17% have mental illness;
- 80% have mental illness among substance misuse population;
- 44% have substance misuse among psychiatric population;
- 40% dual diagnosis in Manchester Mental Health and Social Care Trust.
  Holland & Schulte (2007); Office of National Statistics (2002).

When creating an individual treatment plan for a service user, there are a number of issues that need to be taken into account. These include the rationale for the treatment, especially if there are other issues to consider such as age of service user, previous medicines prescribed, possible risks and benefits. It is important to choose medication on an individual basis, taking note of symptoms and possible interactions with other medicines. Modern medicines have the potential to improve the life of people suffering from many mental health problems. Adherence to an effective regime is a factor that can support the recovery process. Interactions with other medicines must be considered as part of the plan of care in order to minimise any risks to the service user (Flanagan, 2006). It is essential that as a practitioner you familiarise yourself with any possible adverse events and drug interactions that may occur. A role of medicines management is to work with individuals to ensure safe, effective and appropriate use of medicines. A particular problem is the use of medicines outside of their licence, as

Table 3.1 Potential interactions between psychotropic medicines and substances (Alcohol Concern, 2001; Bazire, 2007; Taylor et al., 2007)

	Amphetamines, Ecstasy, cocaine	Cannabis	Opiates	Alcohol	Nicotine
Typical antipsychotics	Opposes antipsychotic effects of chlorpromazine. Haloperidol may moderate stimulant effects. Diminished effect could increase amphetamine use. Flupentixol may reduce craving	Increased metabolism via (cytochrome) CYP450 enzyme induction can lead to increased clearance, e.g. chlorpromazine. Additive drowsiness has been reported	Enhanced sedative and hypotensive effect	No published evidence that alcohol reduces the efficacy of these medicines. The following interactions have been reported: • enhanced central nervous system (CNS) depression • lethargy • hypotension • respiratory depression • drowsiness • may enhance extra-pyramidal side effects and hepatoxicity • chlorpromazine, haloperidol less sedating	Plasma levels of haloperidol 23% lower in smokers. Smokers usually on higher doses of anti-psychotics
Atypical antipsychotics	Atypicals oppose effects of amphetamines and ecstasy. Risperidone may reduce euphoric effect of cocaine but not reduce craving or amount of use. Users may increase use to achieve pre-prescription levels of stimulation. Clozapine increases cocaine levels but reduces high; some cardiac events have been reported	Risk of additive sedation; can reduce serum levels of olanzapine and clozapine via induction of CYP1A2. Clozapine intoxication reported following cessation of cannabis smoking	Case of opiate withdrawal precipitated by risperidone reported	May enhance extra-pyramidal side effects (EPSEs). Increased risk of hypotension and tachycardia with olanzapine. Additive sedation	Olanzapine plasma levels 21% lower in smokers. Faster clearance. Nicotine lowers levels of clozapine. Caution if patient stops smoking or drinking caffeine with clozapine. Lack of interaction shown with smoking and aripiprazole

Table 3.1 *Continued*

	Amphetamines, Ecstasy, cocaine	Cannabis	Opiates	Alcohol	Nicotine
Anticholinergics	Theoretical added effect; increased effect of both	Possible anticholinergic psychosis			Steady-state propranolol levels in smokers reduced via CYP1A2 induction
Anxiolytics and hypnotics	Mutually diminished effect. Amphetamine has reversed sedative and memory-impairing effects of triazolam over sedation	Additive drowsiness Possible paradoxical effect, (glutamate surge) leading to agitation	Dangerous additive sedation (respiratory depression)	Can enhance sedation of benzodiazepines by 20–30% Can also decrease diazepam clearance Buspirone may be safer alternative for people using alcohol Beta-blockers, e.g. propranolol, can accentuate drop in blood pressure and alcohol may reduce absorption and increase clearance Increased bioavailability of clomethiazole Additive CNS effect with chloral hydrate disulfiram-like reaction reported Alcohol's effect of performance impairment is increased by Zaleplon, though short lived	

Lithium	Lithium can oppose effects of amphetamines (suppresses the high) Lithium, ecstasy and over-exercise (dancing) causes dehydration and toxicity Lithium and carbamazepine reduces 'high' of crack cocaine – may prompt users to stop medication	One case report of lithium levels raised to toxic levels when combined with cannabis Additive drowsiness	May produce a 12% increase in peak lithium levels Lithium not sedating Alcohol can dehydrate and increased fluid intake can interfere with lithium
Carbamazepine	Cocaine may enhance the cardiac effects of carbamazepine Carbamazepine leads to increased formation of norcocaine: hepatotoxic and more cardiotoxic than cocaine	Decreases methadone levels; dangerous to stop suddenly The use of sodium valproate is recommended	No published evidence of interaction, but additive sedation should be expected Monitor liver function: LFTs
TCA antidepressants	May reduce cocaine effect Caution: arrhythmias	Marked tachycardia; delirium also reported Selective serotinin re-uptake inhibitor (SSRI) recommended	Additive sedation and hypotension; both lower seizure threshold May affect oral bioavailability of TCAs by reducing first pass metabolism

Table 3.1 *Continued*

	Amphetamines, Ecstasy, Cannabis cocaine	Opiates	Alcohol	Nicotine
SSRI antidepressants	Fluoxetine – increased energy, increased libido, pressured speech; one report of the development of mania after smoking cannabis Amphetamines thought to block serotonin re-uptake hence depressive states Fluoxetine most frequently prescribed with cocaine addiction due to anecdotal anti-craving properties SSRI may increase stimulant toxicity and SSRIs may attenuate psychological effects	Fluvoxamine and possibly paroxetine may increase serum methadone, increase respiratory depression Citalopram opiate neutral Duloxetine sedating	Less sedating than TCA Citalopram and fluoxetine – no significant interactions Fluvoxine may exaggerate effects of alcohol though later study showed no interaction Duloxetine sedating Enhanced sedation noted with mirtazapine	With fluvoxamine there can be a moderately increased side effect experience Fluvoxamine inhibits the metabolism of caffeine and half-life may rise from 5 to 22 h Smoking may lower duloxetine levels by 50%
MAOI antidepressants	Potentially fatal interaction – hypertension, muscle rigidity, vomiting, severe headaches Possibility of hypertension by augmenting pressor effect	Potentially fatal interaction with pethidine	Tyramine, found in wine and beer, can cause dangerous rise in blood pressure after one drink Increased catecholamine release may potentiate alcohol effect	Reports of increased jitteriness with caffeine

unexpected adverse effects may occur due to the unusual usage of a drug. Guidance has been produced to support clinicians in these circumstances (Royal College of Psychiatrists, 2005). Full consent must be obtained when using medicines outside of their licence, which would also include the prescribing of psychotropic medicine at doses above recommended limits.

Substance (mis)use

The question of what is substance use or misuse has been much debated. The questions in Box 3.2 are important to consider when producing a treatment plan with a service user.

The following national guidance is available to guide the clinician:

* National Statistics: Tobacco, alcohol and drug use and mental health. The website link is www.dh.gov.uk/en/Publicationsandstatistics/Publications/PublicationsPolicyAndGuidance/DH_062649
* Mental health policy implementation guide: Dual diagnosis good practice guide. The website link is www.dh.gov.uk/en/Publicationsandstatistics/Publications/PublicationsPolicy-AndGuidance/DH_4009058

Substance use/misuse appears to be prevalent in up to 44% of the adult population admitted with mental health issues. In these situations, any substance use has the potential to hinder the initial assessment, treatment and possible recovery from 'mental ill health' (Department of Health, 2006b). Alongside the diagnosis of mental illness any co-morbid substance use will have a major impact on any effective treatment. Research suggests that there are various substances that can have a profound effect on the individual. Opioids, by nature, are highly addictive and opioid dependence is a chronic relapsing

---

Box 3.2 Substance mis(use)

* What is substance use?
* What is substance misuse?
* How do we classify what is 'use' and 'misuse'?
* When does using substances become a problem?
* What effect does substance use have on service users with mental health problems?
* What is the percentage of substance use in the mental health setting?

disorder (O'Shea et al., 2006). When this is considered alongside an individual who has what society classes as a 'lifetime illness' then it is clear that co-morbid substance use can often have a detrimental effect on the recovery of the individual.

Safe prescribing and management of the service user with a dual diagnosis

It is clear from the above that at least 40% of service users suffering from a mental illness will be using other non-prescribed substances. Many will also smoke tobacco. There is limited published information available to guide the prescriber on how to prescribe safely when aware that other substances are also being consumed. It is also unlikely that any robust research will be conducted into this area. Tables 3.1 and 3.2

Table 3.2 A guide to support prescribing decisions when advising a service user quitting smoking. From Bazire (2007) and Taylor *et al.* (2007)

	Effect of stopping smoking on drug	Dosing advice
Haloperidol	Plasma levels may rise by 23%	Haloperidol dose may need to be decreased
Clozapine	Plasma levels may increase by 72%	Decrease dose
Olanzapine	Increased by 21%	May need to decrease dose
Fluvoxamine	Increase plasma levels	May need to decrease dose
Propranolol	Increased plasma levels	May need to decrease dose
Duloxetine	Plasma levels may increase by 50%	May need to decrease dose
Fluphenazine	Plasma levels may increase	Monitor symptoms/side effects
Beta-blockers	Plasma levels may increase	Review dose
Flecainide	Increased plasma level	May need to decrease dose
Insulin	Plasma levels may increase when stopping smoking	Review dose of insulin and monitor blood glucose
Theophylline/aminophylline	Increased plasma levels	Decrease dose by 25–33% within 1 week of stopping smoking Monitor patient as further alterations in dosage may be required
Cimetidine	Nicotine increases cimetidine levels	May need to decrease cimetidine dose or use alternative H_2 antagonist, e.g. ranitidine

are an attempt to summarise the current literature and research. The aim is to provide a guide for clinicians and to start collecting information on a more widespread basis. Only further qualitative, practice-based research can help in identifying which interactions are truly relevant to the service user.

Possible interactions between psychotropic agents and non-prescribed drugs

It is necessary to consider the issues in Box 3.3 when producing a treatment plan for a service user.

It is important to remember that non-prescribed medicines can come from a variety of sources and may be licensed products. They are not all illicit substances. There are many over-the-counter medicines that the individual can use to 'self-medicate'. Non-prescribed drugs can also be accessed from friends and family, through the internet or countries with different licensing regulations. This increased availability means that individuals can 'self-prescribe' products to manage their symptoms. These products include many prescription only medicines (POMs) that would normally only be available from qualified prescribers.

Antipsychotics reduce the psychotropic effect of almost all drugs of abuse by blocking dopamine receptors (dopamine is the neurotransmitter responsible for reward). Patients prescribed antipsychotics may increase their consumption of illicit substances to compensate for this blockage.

Tricyclic antidepressants are known to potentiate the effect of opiates. This in turn can lead to the potential for respiratory depression. If antidepressants are prescribed, it is advisable to avoid those which

---

Box 3.3   Consideration for developing a treatment plan

- What are the non-prescribed drugs that the service user may be using in addition to those prescribed?
- What are the potential problems with these non-prescribed substances? (This would include whether these were legal and what risk the service user was facing in accessing and administering these substances.)
- What are the reported and possible interactions with the non-prescribed drugs?
- Formulate a clinical judgement regarding how interactions between all the substances, medicines and any co-morbid conditions and personal conditions may adversely affect the service user.

cause sedation, especially where a person consumes high amounts of alcohol.

The potential to induce respiratory depression is also present for people taking antipsychotic medicines, therefore preparations with increased levels of sedation as a side effect should be avoided by people who use high amounts of alcohol.

In this section the substances discussed will be those used most commonly with the greatest amount of evidence.

Cannabis

The prevalence of cannabis misuse varies across the age range. Two-thirds of substance misusers under the age of 18 years who are in treatment report that cannabis is their drug of choice; this use is often associated with increased use of alcohol (Department of Health (England) and the devolved administrations, 2007). There are reported interactions with cannabis and both physical and psychotropic medicines. Table 3.1 highlights some of the risks when cannabis is taken with psychotropic medication.

Opiates

When opiates are taken with other 'drugs or substances' there is the potential for an interaction. Medicines and substances that are used to depress the central nervous system (CNS), i.e. benzodiazepines, tricyclic antidepressants and alcohol, have been known to increase CNS depression, which may lead to the probability of respiratory depression (the slowing or cessation of an individual's breathing). The evidence suggests that all opiates have the potential for this effect. Table 3.1 identifies possible interactions between prescribed psychotropic agents and opiates. Certain physical health medicines also have the potential to interact with opioids, although not all opioids are affected. Some of these medicines decrease opioid levels whilst others can act as partial agonists. When methadone is used with opioid antagonists, such as naltrexone or naloxone, there is potential for withdrawal symptoms if methadone has recently been taken. With medicines that may decrease opioid levels, i.e. carbamazepine, HIV medicines and St John's wort, the dose of methadone or buprenorphine may need to be increased to prevent withdrawal symptoms (Department of Health (England) and the devolved administrations, 2007).

Stimulants

Research suggests that treatment for people who abuse stimulants is best offered in the form of psychosocial and non-pharmacological interventions. Pharmacological agents have been tried for treatment of withdrawal but there does not appear to be enough evidence to suggest that pharmacological treatments are effective, particularly in promoting abstinence. It appears that giving advice about safe techniques, and preventative measures to minimise risks associated with stimulant use, are more effective (Department of Health (England) and the devolved administrations, 2007).

There is little documented evidence of interactions with hallucinogens (LSD, magic mushrooms, and mescaline).

Alcohol

Similar to the issues raised for non-prescribed medicines it is important to remember the issues listed in Box 3.4 when considering treatment options for service users using alcohol. See Table 3.1 for potential interactions alcohol may have with prescribed medicines.

Nicotine

The issue of interactions with medicines and smoking has been discussed previously but the questions in Box 3.5 need to be considered.

In 2002, a national survey was carried out looking at tobacco, alcohol and other drug use, and their relationship to psychiatric morbidity (Office of National Statistics, 2002). The survey focused on adults between the ages of 16 and 74 years. The survey results, focusing on nicotine use, showed that smokers were more likely than non-smokers to:

- be younger (those aged 16–24 were nearly six times more likely to be smokers than the oldest age group, once other factors had been taken into account);
- be cohabiting, divorced or separated rather than married (42, 41 and 23%, respectively, were current smokers);

Box 3.4   Issues to be considered regarding alcohol

- Safe drinking limits and advice on units of alcohol.
- Chemical components of alcohol and how these components act on brain chemistry.
- Alcohol and mental health medication.
- Alcohol and combined use in mental health.
- What effect does this have on mood?
- What changes need to be made to the medication?

Box 3.5   Issues to be considered with smokers

- Population of mental health patients who smoke?
- Smoking cessation services and support, including availability of a range of different NRT products?
- Interactions between smoking, smoking cessation and various medicines?
- Physical health and smoking?

- have fewer qualifications (for example, 22% of people with qualification of A level standard or above reported current smoking compared with 32% of those with GCSE level only and 36% of those with no qualifications).

Other factors associated with smoking were being unemployed, working in a manual occupation, having lower household income, being in financial difficulty and living in an urban area (Office of National Statistics, 2002).

Smoking and interactions with medication

Many medicines are broken down by the liver using enzymes belonging to the cytochrome P450 group. If a substance induces or inhibits one of these enzymes then it can affect the dose of a drug that needs to be given to a patient. There are over 3000 chemicals in cigarette smoke but it is not known which ones are significant with regard to drug interactions. Cigarette smoke is a potent inducer of the cytochrome P450 1A2 isoenzyme. Various medications are metabolised using this enzyme and therefore may be affected if a patient starts or stops smoking. Table 3.2 lists the medications that could be affected by a patient stopping smoking.

In mental health services the interactions with clozapine are the most significant. Abruptly stopping smoking when taking clozapine can lead to large increases in clozapine plasma levels and a range of adverse effects. These adverse effects have been serious, such as suffering a seizure. The majority of mental health services supply clozapine through secondary care, owing to the blood testing and licensing agreements for clozapine. However, the service user may be well and being cared for in primary care. It is important that good shared care arrangements are in place to ensure that primary care are aware of the risk of changing smoking habits without discussing possible effects on clozapine levels with the service user, carer and care team.

Pharmacological management

Pharmacological management is addressed in many different pieces of national guidance. National Institute of Clinical Excellence (NICE) guidance and the National Treatment Agency (NTA) have produced the following:

- NICE (www.nice.org.uk)
- NTA (www.nta.nhs.uk/publications/documents/clinical_guidelines_2007)

Physical co-morbidity

There are many co-morbid conditions that affect service users with a severe mental illness more commonly than the general population. These conditions can affect the way medicines are best used and the choice of each medicine. Supporting the physical health needs of people with a severe mental illness has become a government priority because of the range of conditions more prevalent in this group and the range of adverse effects experienced. More information can be found by accessing the *Choosing Health* document, available on the Department of Health website (Department of Health, 2006a).

Liver/kidney disease

When considering drug interactions, the roles of the liver and kidney are crucial to the ability of the body to process substances. Any disorder of the liver or kidneys can lead to interactions, adverse reactions or changes to the general handling of any medicines ingested.

Case study

The case study in Box 3.6 is an example of issues that may occur with service users who may experience potential interactions between pre-scribed medicines and illicit substances.

Conclusion

Many interactions are harmless or theoretical rather than a major concern clinically. The severity of each interaction varies greatly between individuals, with certain groups such as older people being at higher risk of interactions due to being on multiple medicines and complicated regimes, as well as also having co-morbid conditions. Interactions may be advantageous, with the clinician using the

Box 3.6   Case study of interactions

The following questions will need to be addressed whilst reading this case study:

1.   What issues should the clinician consider?
2.   What interactions may occur?
3.   If medication changes are required, how these should be initiated?

Mr M.B. is a 34-year-old man with a dual diagnosis of bipolar disorder complicated by poly-substance abuse.

His current prescribed medication is as follows:

- lithium carbonate (Priadel™) 1.2 g at night
- carbamazepine (Tegretol™) 400 mg twice daily
- olanzapine (Zyprexa™) 15 mg at night
- methadone liquid (1 mg in 1 ml) 60 ml daily
- diazepam (Valium™) 2–5 mg when required

Medication is generally prescribed by his general practitioner (GP) and he is asked to attend the surgery every 3 months for blood monitoring. Mr M.B. does not always attend these appointments. He is also under the care of a consultant psychiatrist and receives an outpatient appointment every 9–12 months.

Mr M.B. obtains his medication from a local pharmacy via a monthly repeat prescription sent to the pharmacy from the GP. He collects methadone from the same pharmacy via a prescription from the Drug and Alcohol Team. Consumption of his methadone is supervised by the pharmacist. He also buys codeine linctus from various other pharmacies for a 'tickly cough' (two pharmacies have now refused him).

Mr M.B. regularly obtains illicit supplies of diazepam and lorazepam, which he uses in addition to his prescribed dose. He drinks alcohol quite heavily when he 'feels stressed' – usually strong lager and vodka or whisky. He previously smoked a lot of cannabis but has recently cut down and prefers to use alcohol or 'benzos' to relax. He hardly ever smokes tobacco alone.

Mr M.B. recently started to feel excessively tired and drowsy which he attributed to his medication. He felt generally unwell and was feeling nauseous and occasionally vomited. He decided to stop his olanzapine, lithium and carbamazepine to see if that made him feel better. He stopped vomiting but continued to feel worse over the next couple of weeks and was very lethargic. He thought it might be because he 'needed cannabis' and took more diazepam to relax.

He was found unconscious in his garden by a neighbour, who called an ambulance.

Summary of interactions

Methadone + other CNS depressants
Additive or synergistic effect greatly increases the risk of overdose and potential for developing fatal respiratory depression.

Alcohol + benzodiazepines, e.g. diazepam and or other opiates
Combination of alcohol/benzodiazepines with methadone is one of the main causes of fatal overdose.

Olanzapine and interactions
Olanzapine is metabolised in the liver by enzymes (CYP1A2).
   Chemicals in tobacco smoke 'induce' this enzyme making blood levels lower.
   Stopping smoking tobacco (or cannabis) causes olanzapine levels to rise.
   This may add to the sedation he has been feeling.

Methadone + carbamazepine
Methadone has a long half-life and as a result it can take an extended period to be removed from the body. As a consequence, toxicity can be cumulative, occurring over a period of time.
   The drug is mainly metabolised in the liver by one of the cytochrome P450 enzymes. Carbamazepine is an 'inducer' of this enzyme system and as a result methadone is removed more quickly.
   When carbamazepine is stopped, the enzyme is no longer induced and methadone is removed more slowly, causing methadone blood levels rise.
   This combination with benzodiazepines + alcohol causes excessive CNS depression, possibly resulting in unconsciousness + respiratory depression, which can possibly be fatal.

Lithium and interactions
Lithium blood levels need to be very carefully controlled as there is a narrow 'therapeutic window' and a slight increase in levels can be toxic.
   Alcohol use may cause dehydration and, as a result, the excretion of lithium can become inhibited, causing blood levels to rise.
   Relapse of mania may result fairly quickly after stopping anti-manic drugs especially lithium.

Cannabis and interactions
Cannabis may cause lithium levels to rise, causing toxicity. Stopping cannabis may cause levels to fall and leading to relapse.
   Cannabis + olanzapine increases drowsiness/sedation and can reduce the efficacy of the antipsychotic.
   Cannabis + benzodiazepines increases drowsiness and can increase agitation and edginess.

Continued

Summary

Methadone, alcohol, olanzapine, lithium, benzodiazepines, carbamazepine, codeine, and cannabis all contribute to sedation and respiratory depression.

- Carbamazepine keeps methadone plasma levels lower.
- Smoking keeps olanzapine plasma levels lower.
- Cannabis increases lithium blood levels.
- Alcohol increases lithium blood levels.

Case study kindly provided by Karen Bennett, senior mental health pharmacist, Manchester Mental Health & Social care Trust, Central Manchester.

interaction to change plasma levels of medicines and achieve required outcomes. It is important, however, to note that the information currently available is limited and speculative and further research and practice-based work is required before this important area is fully understood.

References

Alcohol Concern (2001) *Dangerous Cocktails. Your Mental Health Medication and Alcohol. What are the Facts?* Fact Sheet 3. Alcohol Concern, London.

Bazire, S. (2007) *Psychotropic Drug Directory: The Professionals' Pocket Handbook and Aide Memoire.* Crownwell Press, Wiltshire.

Department of Health. (2006a) *Choosing Health: Supporting the Physical Health Needs of people with Severe Mental Illness Commissioning Framework.* HMSO, London.

Department of Health (2006b) *Dual Diagnosis in Mental Health Inpatient and Day Hospital Settings – Guidance on the Assessment and Management of Patients in Mental Health Inpatient and Day Hospital Settings who have Mental Ill-Health and Substance Use Problems.* HMSO, London.

Department of Health (England) and the devolved administrations. (2007) *Drug Misuse and Dependence: UK Guidelines on Clinical Management.* Department of Health (England), the Scottish Government, Welsh Assembly Government and Northern Ireland Executive, London.

Drugs and Therapeutics Bulletin (2007) How safe are antipsychotics in dementia? *Drugs and Therapeutics Bulletin,* **45**(11), 81–84.

Flanagan, R. (2006) Therapeutic monitoring of antipyschotic drugs. *CPD Clinical Biochemistry,* **7**(1), 3–18.

Holland, M. & Schulte, S. (2008) Dual diagnosis in Manchester, UK: practitioners' estimates of prevalence rates in mental health and substance misuse services. *Mental Health and Substance Use: Dual Diagnosis,* **1**(2), 118–124.

Joint Formulary Committee (2008) *British National Formulary*. British Medical Association and Royal Pharmaceutical Society of Great Britain, London.

O'Shea, J., Law, F. & Melichar, J. (2006) Opioid dependence. *BMJ Clinical Evidence*, web publication date 01 June 2007.

Office of National Statistics (2002) *National Statistics: Tobacco, Alcohol and Drug Use and Mental Health*. HMSO, London.

Royal College of Psychiatrists (2005) *Use of Licensed Medicines for Unlicensed Applications in Psychiatric Practice*. Royal College of Psychiatrists, London.

Taylor, D., Paton, C. & Kerwin, R. (2007) *The Maudsley Prescribing Guidelines 2006–2007*. Taylor and Francis Group, London.

www.dh.gov.uk/en/Publicationsandstatistics/Publications/Publications-PolicyAndGuidance/DH_062649. Accessed 16/09/08.

www.dh.gov.uk/en/Publicationsandstatistics/Publications/Publications-PolicyAndGuidance/DH_4009058. Accessed 16/09/08.

Part 2

Medicines management in clinical practice

Non-medical prescribing and medicines management policies

Alison Hay, Steve Hemingway and Steven Jones

Introduction

The appropriate use of medicines when used in combination with other therapies has a lot to offer service users receiving care and treatment. One of the challenges facing clinicians is selecting appropriate pharmacotherapy to ensure that service users gain the best possible outcome from their medicine. This is more complex than merely selecting a particular drug; it takes into account the evidence base for decision-making and ensures that service users are fully engaged as partners in treatment decisions.

Medicines management, including changes to prescriptive authority through developments around non-medical prescribing and to the regulations for controlled drugs, have formed part of the UK Government's agenda to modernise health service provision (Department of Health, 2000).

Choice and flexibility in care and treatment decisions are the key ingredients of a modernised healthcare service. Non-medical prescribing in mental health is one such development that increases service user choice (Jones & Jones, 2008) and also provides access to treatments in a timely manner (Nolan & Bradley, 2007).

Non-medical prescribing – the background

Non-medical prescribing is an umbrella term that is used to describe professional groups that are permitted to prescribe medicines but who do not fall under the professional group of doctors, dentists and veterinarians. There are many different ways in which non-medical prescribers may prescribe medicines. This is largely dependent upon which profession they belong to, when they completed their training and what medicines they are seeking to prescribe.

The Acts enabling non-medical prescribing

The *Medicines Act 1968*, although nearly four decades old, is still the legislation that regulates the prescribing of medicines. The Act restricts the prescribing of prescription only medicines to 'appropriate practitioners', originally deemed to be doctors, dentists and veterinarians. The *Medicines Act* was amended by the *Medicinal Products: prescription by Nurses Act 1992* to allow nurses to prescribe from a limited formulary. There was, however, a requirement for this to be followed by amendments to the Pharmaceutical Services Regulations 1994 to enable pharmacists to dispense prescriptions that were written by nurses. The limited formulary was subsequently followed by the development of extended and supplementary modes of prescribing for nurses (Department of Health, 2001) and was enabled in law by the *Health and Social Care Act 2001*, allowing appropriately qualified nurses, pharmacists and allied health professionals in mental health care to prescribe medications within their scope of practice. The legal framework for non-medical prescribing is shown in Box 4.1.

Box 4.1   Legal framework for the development of non-medical prescribing

Medicines Act 1968 and *Dangerous Drugs Act 1972*

   Medicinal Products: prescription by Nurses Act 1992
   Pharmaceutical Services Regulations 1994
   Health and Social Care Act 2001
   Misuse of Drugs Act 1971 modification order 2001
   Mental Capacity Act 2005
   Misuse of Drugs Act alterations 2005
   The Prescription Only Medicines (Human Use) Amendment Order 2008

Developments in non-medical prescribing

Limited formulary nurse prescribing

Limited formulary nurse prescribing commenced initially with a pilot study and was rolled out nationally in 1998. The first generation of non-medical prescribers able to use the limited formulary in the UK were community nurses (district nurses and health visitors) who, after training, were permitted to prescribe a small number of items, mainly consisting of dressings for wound care but also included general sales list, pharmacy and a few prescription only medicines.

Extended formulary nurse prescribing

In 2002, nurses who successfully completed a programme of training and registered with the Nursing and Midwifery Council (NMC) were permitted to prescribe for a range of medical conditions using an extended nurse prescribing formulary. Initially, prescribing was restricted to one of four key areas: health promotion, minor injuries, minor ailments and palliative care. Despite additions to the extended nurse prescribing formulary in 2002, it was clear that the relevance to mental health was limited.

Supplementary prescribing

An opportunity arose in 2003 for UK mental health nurses (who had successfully completed the appropriate course and registered with the NMC) to prescribe medicines from the *British National Formulary* (*BNF*), including psychotropic medication, as part of a 'supplementary pre-scribing' arrangement. This initially excluded controlled drugs, but amendments to the *Misuse of Drugs Act 2001* in April 2005 removed restrictions placed on the medicines that are permitted to be included within a clinical management plan (CMP), with the exclusion of Schedule One drugs (Box 4.2).

Supplementary prescribing is defined as a voluntary partnership between a doctor (or dentist) and a qualified supplementary prescriber to develop a plan of care around the use of medicines to treat a specific individual for a specific condition.

The initial diagnosis is required to be completed by the doctor (or dentist) and then a plan of care, the CMP, is drawn up with the service user's agreement once an initial diagnosis is completed by the doctor (or dentist). The CMP is intended to be a specific plan that is unique

---

Box 4.2   Schedule One drugs

Includes drugs such as cannabis and lysergide, which are not used medicinally. Possession and supply are prohibited except in accordance with Home Office authority.

Joint Formulary Committee (2008)

Table 4.1 Condition to be treated: depression

Broad clinical management plan	Specific clinical management plan
Any SSRI medication within the dosing schedule listed in the BNF (2008) Not exceeding maximum doses	Escitalopram 10 mg once a day for 14 days and then increase to 20 mg once a day

for each individual and details the condition(s) and treatment(s) that are to be included under the supplementary prescribing arrangement. This is a significant development, enabling the prescribing of the service user's medication, including controlled drugs to be added to the medications that non-medical prescribers are permitted to prescribe. Clinical management plans can vary hugely in their content, not least in that they are individually written for each service user but in that they may be broad-based or very specific (or somewhere in between). For example, a broad-based CMP may just state the condition to be treated and suggest a group type of medicine within the limits of the BNF (Joint Formulary Committee (2008). A specific plan may detail the condition to be treated and state the medicine to be prescribed; see Table 4.1 for a broad and a specific CMP for depression.

Each plan is required to detail any specific limitations and restrictions to supplementary prescribing and include information on when the pharmacological management should be referred back to the independent prescriber (doctor/dentist). In addition, the plan should also include details of arrangements for notifying any adverse incidents. With the addition of controlled drugs, all prescribing clinicians need to be mindful of the ramifications of the Harold Shipman case, which clearly highlights the legal and ethical issues associated with prescriptive practice and the need to work within the parameters of the law (www.the-shipman-inquiry.org.uk/home.asp).

Independent nurse prescribing

In 2006 legislation was passed that permitted appropriately qualified nurses to prescribe any medication licensed for use as detailed in the BNF (Joint Formulary Committee, 2008). Guidance recommended that this was required to be in the scope of the nurses' professional practice and clinical competency (Department of Health, 2006b). Such development gave a real opportunity for mental health nurses to expand upon their experiences as supplementary prescribers and to make independent decisions in conjunction with service users regarding medication. Unlike supplementary prescribing, independent prescribing enables the nurse to assess, diagnose and formulate a treatment plan independently from a doctor (Wix, 2007; Jones, 2008). There are also develop-

---

Box 4.3 Case example – Independent and supplementary prescribing

Ellie Gordon, a nurse prescriber who specialises in addiction, works primarily with service users who are dependent upon opiates and require maintenance prescribing of controlled drugs. She is required to have a good awareness, not only of the pharmacology of the main prescribed drugs of methadone and buprenorphine, but also to keep up to date with the prescribing of controlled drugs in a post-Shipman era. She requires a good working knowledge of medications relating to mental health issues such as depression and anxiety, as well as an awareness of basic wound care and nutrition prescribing. This means that the range of information that is obtained and sourced needs to be wide and varied in nature; this includes signing up for email alerts from statutory organisations linked to these areas of prescribing such as the National Prescribing Centre, Department of Health and the Royal College of Nursing (RCN) clinical governance bulletin. Doing so has contributed to Ellie's ability to remain up to date and contributes to her prescribing in a safe and efficient manner, both as a supplementary and as an independent prescriber.

Adapted from Gordon (2006)

Box 4.4 Summary of developments

1994 – Limited formulary prescribing (frequently referred to as V100)
2002 – Extended formulary prescribing (frequently referred to as V200)
2003 – Supplementary prescribing
2005 – Supplementary prescribers able to prescribe controlled drugs
2006 – Independent prescribers able to prescribe any licensed medicine (except controlled drugs)
2008 – The independent prescribing of all controlled drugs

---

ments that will enable mental health nurses to prescribe controlled drugs independently (Risk Review, 2008). An example of independent and supplementary prescribing is shown in Box 4.3, and a summary of the developments in prescribing is shown in Box 4.4.

Future prescribing developments

There have been significant developments in relation to non-medical prescribing and other professional groups, for example pharmacists, have their own prescribing formularies and there are developments to run clinics and offer additional treatments in pharmacies (Department of Health, 2008). In addition, there is an increasing list of allied health professionals (AHP) who are permitted to supplementary prescribe (www.npc.co.uk), thus making better use of practitioners' skills and knowledge through adopting new ways of working (Department of Health, 2006a;2007).

Patient group directions

Changes that occurred in August 2000 to medicines legislation clarified the law in relation to the supplying or administration of medicines under patient group directions (PGDs) (Nursing and Midwifery Council, 2004). Patient group directions are not a form of prescribing but are a form of supplying and administering medicines to a specified group of people who may not have been identified prior to presenting for treatment. Typical examples where PGDs are used is in the area of primary care and walk-in centres where vaccinations/immunisations may be administered or contraceptive medicine supplied without an individual prescription being required.

The process of developing PGDs can be complex, involving a multi-disciplinary team and the local drug and therapeutics committee. Patient group directions are required to be formally authorised through clinical governance mechanisms, with trusts or healthcare organisations needing clear policies about who can supply and administer medicines under a PGD and under what circumstances. To date PGDs have not been widely adopted in the area of mental health practice. There are, however, examples emerging of some mental health services using PGDs (see Box 4.5). A resource to support the development of PGDs can be found through the National Electronic Library for Medicines (NeLM) (www.portal.nelm.nhs.uk/PGD/default.aspx).

Box 4.5   Case example – Patient group directions

Patient group directions (PGDs) in crisis/home treatment teams have enabled nursing staff to offer immediate treatment to service users experiencing sleeping difficulties, high levels of agitation/anxiety or extra-pyramidal side effects. Algorithms to support appropriate use have been developed.

Adapted from National Prescribing Centre (2005)

Prescribing and supplying medicines in practice

In practice, different professions may be prescribing or administering medicines to service users through a variety of methods that may

> **Box 4.6   Case example – Service level agreements**
>
> A mental health NHS Trust set up service level agreements with local primary care trusts (PCTs) enabling non-medical prescribers employed by the mental health trust to prescribe in neighbouring PCTs. Under these arrangements the non-medical prescribers used policies and procedures in the Trust that they are prescribing in and had separate prescription pads.
>
> Adapted from National Prescribing Centre (2005)

involve prescribing formularies, supplementary prescribing CMPs or PGDs. For example, in mental health, antipsychotic medication may be prescribed as part of a supplementary prescribing CMP, a laxative may be prescribed from a prescribing formulary and an analgesic may be prescribed through PGDs. The non-medical prescriber would, in this instance, be using three distinctly different methods of prescribing practice or supplying/administering medicine. This presents challenges for all involved to have an appreciation of the way in which medicines are being prescribed or supplied, and the opportunities and restrictions that are placed upon prescribing practice. Box 4.6 gives a case example of service level agreements.

With the increasing emphasis on meeting the physical health needs of those in contact with mental health services (Department of Health, 2006a; Healthcare Commission, 2007), it is more likely that mental health practitioners will be prescribing a broad range of different medicines. This may be increased when addressing the needs of those presenting with dual diagnoses (for example, administering hepatitis B vaccinations), health promotion strategies (smoking cessation, nutritional supplements, contraceptives) and co-morbidities associated with long-term health conditions and disease prevention strategies, for example heart disease and diabetes (Nash, 2005).

Non-medical prescribers will need to ensure that they have the support of their employing organisation, the agreement of the service user and ultimately the competency to prescribe or to administer medication through a PGD (National Prescribing Centre, 2001; Jones, 2008; Bradley et al., 2007).

Competency in non-medical prescribing

Competency is an area often raised by non-medical prescribers and organisations (Hay et al., 2004; Hemingway, 2004; Jones, 2008). In expanding their role, non-medical prescribers must be clear about their accountability for determining how they remain up to date and whether

---

Box 4.7 Case example – Competency

A learning need around psychopharmacology was identified by nurses working in a mental health trust who had completed the non-medical prescribing course. In response to this the Trust commissioned, through their local higher education institution (HEI), additional courses around psychopharmacology. All nurses were actively encouraged to undertake the training as part of their continuing professional development.

Adapted from Skingsley et al. (2006)

---

they possess the necessary knowledge, skills and competence to prescribe. In addition, non-medical prescribers need to understand the nature of tasks and responsibilities associated with the development of new clinical roles, such as non-medical prescribing, upon working relationships and the clinical environment (Hay et al., 2004; Bradley et al., 2007). The National Prescribing Centre publishes information to support and guide non-medical prescribers and organisations in identifying ongoing professional development needs (www.npc.co.uk/non_medical.htm). Box 4.7 gives a case example of competency in prescribing.

Peer support, particularly in the initial stages of prescribing practice, is absolutely essential (Jukes et al., 2004). Otway (2002) identified that non-medical prescribers who did not receive support from their peers and team members were often discouraged from prescribing. Those who did not prescribe soon after qualifying often lost confidence (Baird, 2004). Confidence is an essential factor which affects the non-medical prescriber's decision to use his or her prescriptive skills, with the level of confidence being correlated with the level of prescribing practice (While & Biggs, 2004, Bradley et al., 2008). A case example of peer support is shown in Box 4.8.

Box 4.8 Case example – Support

Monthly peer group supervision sessions were made mandatory in one NHS Trust to support nurses in their role. These sessions initially involved problem-based learning scenarios (i.e. video clips, case scenarios, etc.) as triggers for discussion in the supervision session. As the nurses' role developed, and more complex cases formed part of the nurses' prescribing experience, the problem-based learning 'triggers' were replaced with real-life scenarios and dilemmas.

Adapted from Hay (2005)

The legal and ethical issues of non-medical prescribing

Non-maleficence and beneficence are two ethical issues surrounding prescribing practice. Non-maleficence refers to not inflicting harm and beneficence refers to removing harm and promoting good (Foster, 2002). It is both the legal and professional duty of the nurse in mental health care to prescribe in a mode that facilitates beneficent interventions.

Reasonable and responsible non-medical prescribers, by law, should work in a way where no harm is done to the service user and within their scope of practice (Nursing and Midwifery Council, 2008). The Bolam 'principle' or 'test' was established by the *Bolam v Friern Barnet Hospital Management Committee (1957)* (Kennedy & Grubb, 2000). A medical practitioner, for example, is not negligent if he or she acts in accordance with a practice accepted at the time as proper by a responsible body of medical opinion, for which medical and non-medical prescribers will be measured against the practices of a 'reasonable other' professional when called to account for their practice.

With the advent of non-medical prescribing being a recent event, there has been no test of the Bolam principle but it is, nevertheless, of significant relevance. The use of the Bolam test has been criticised as not relevant to modern day services as it allows the medical profession to state the standard on which they will be judged. More recently the courts have refined Bolam, and that the judge should decide in the case of negligence, as outlined in *Bolitho v Hackney Health Authority 1997* (Foster, 2002). The Bolitho case established that even though there may be more than one course of action, the course chosen must withstand logical analysis. Practitioners therefore may have more than one option, but must be able to justify the course that they adopted. Negligence has been defined as:

> *'the omission to do something which a reasonable man, guided upon these conditions which ordinarily regulate the conduct of human affairs would do or something which a prudent and reasonable man would not do'*
>
> *Blyth v Birmingham Water Works (1856)*

The responsible or reasonable non-medical prescriber owes service users a duty of care. This duty entails taking care and practising to a standard that ensures that, as far as reasonably practicable, service users are not caused harm or damage. If however, this duty of care is breached and the service user can prove that any subsequent harm or damage is due to the breach and that the harm was reasonably foreseeable, then he or she has a right to sue for negligence (Gibson, 2001).

The extra responsibility associated with prescribing brings with it increased accountability. Fletcher (2000) comments on the 'compensationalist' culture where society sees a financial opportunity and encourages suing. If mistakes in healthcare interventions occur then nurses may in the future find themselves more directly involved in civil proceedings. It is an increasing feature that under common law, courts are willing to hear cases brought by individuals or organisations that wish to challenge the decision of a public body or for clarification when no legislation exists (Caulfield, 1999). To date there has been no use of this law regarding non-medical prescribing. It is, however, likely to feature in the future. It is therefore paramount that the nurse is both knowledgeable of, and practises within, the law, as ignorance is no defence (Gibson, 2001).

Consent

In law, any adult who is mentally competent (i.e. has capacity) has the right to consent to or refuse their treatment (Gibson, 2001). Any non-consensual touching could result in a civil action for trespass to the person. Consent can be implied, for example they roll up their sleeve when blood is about to be taken for clozaril screening, or expressed, for example when consent is given verbally or in writing. Non-medical prescribers need to be aware of their professional and legal responsibility for giving appropriate and sufficient information, on which a balanced judgement of whether to accept or refuse the treatment can be made.

Of particular relevance to prescribing in mental health care is the case when the service user is incapable of giving a valid consent, then the *Mental Capacity Act 2005* (www.dca.gov.uk/menincap/bill-summary.htm) places a statutory duty on the health professional to act in the best interests of his or her client following the five key principles of the Act (Dimond, 2008), namely:

- a presumption of capacity – every adult has the right to make his or her own decisions and must be assumed to have capacity to do so unless it is proved otherwise;
- the right for individuals to be supported to make their own decisions – people must be given all appropriate help before anyone concludes that they cannot make their own decisions;
- that individuals must retain the right to make what might be seen as eccentric or unwise decisions;
- best interests – anything done for or on behalf of people without capacity must be in their best interests and

- least restrictive intervention – anything done for or on behalf of people without capacity should be the least restrictive of their basic rights and freedoms.

It is a matter of good practice that the prescribing professional should consult with close relatives or significant others to obtain their assent; this should then be recorded in the notes. Under the *Mental Health Act (MHA) 1983*, where treatment can be given without the service user's consent, may be too complex a scenario for the non-medical prescriber in the supplementary prescribing role. However, Mazhindu and Brownsell (2003) speculate that as the *Mental Health Amendments Act 2007* becomes law the non-medical prescriber could act in the service user's 'best interest' in the community setting where a community treatment order of the amended Act has been applied, giving them authority to prescribe, treat and administer drug therapy for service users under their care. Specific guidance from the professional bodies and local employing organisation will be crucial in this domain.

Finally, and essentially, all professionals working in healthcare should have a reasonable working knowledge of the *Mental Capacity Act (MCA) 2005*, which that provides a decision-making framework for staff to work within for those who may lack the capacity to consent to the treatment at that time and attempting to establish if treatment is necessary and in the clients' best interests. The interface between the MCA and the MHA is a considerable topical debate area; we therefore advise professionals to take each case and situation individually, and taking the least restrictive option that is applicable and marries this to the option that is in the client's best interests. We strongly urge all non-medical prescribers to read wider in relation to the MCA 2005 (Dimond, 2008).

If the client has a contemporaneous advance directive then this refusal has to be seriously considered, and when the circumstances closely match then they should be respected. They must also be contemporary within the lasting power of attorney (LPA) for health and welfare. If they have appointed an attorney under the LPA personal welfare, then this attorney may consent on the patient's behalf if the person lacks capacity for the particular decision at that moment in time. Details of the LPA or advanced refusal are best obtained in advance of the situation arising and the clinical team must be fully aware of their course of action and legal duty. Legal advice may be required for such eventualities. The blanket phrase of 'he or she lacks capacity' should be immediately challenged by 'lacks capacity for what?' at that moment in time. Box 4.9 gives a case example of the issues surrounding capacity.

Box 4.9   Case example – Capacity

Margaret Smith, senior sister at the memory clinic in Doncaster, prescribes acetylcholinesterase medication for service users in the early stages of Alzheimer's disease. Margaret qualified as a supplementary prescriber in September 2003 and in the intervening 18 months actively prepared herself to be knowledgeable regarding the law which she would practise within, combined with formal supervision arrangements and local clinical governance frameworks. When preparing for the prescribing role Margaret in particular sought guidance on consent issues where there may be issues of the service users' ability to give valid consent. When capacity is questioned she seeks appropriate legal advice.

Adapted from Smith and Hemmingway (2005)

Vicarious liability

In reality, clinical staff are indemnified in respect of their NHS employing organisation. That means that even if there were a successful claim for damages against a non-medical prescriber, the employing organisation would pay those damages without recourse to recover damages from the individual prescriber (Preece, 2002). However, any individual who prescribes medication outside of his or her scope of practice or expertise, for example a supplementary prescriber prescribing a drug to treat a condition which is not on the CMP and harm occurs to the service user as a result, then vicarious liability of the employer would not hold in this case. Essentially, the prescriber's job description and contract should also specify this expectation to prescribe non-medically.

Medicines management policy

Medicines management forms part of an organisation's clinical governance responsibility in ensuring the effective use of medicines. This involves the judicious, safe, appropriate and effective use of medicines (Weekes et al., 2005). Medicines management policies must comply with the *Medicine Act 1968* and the *Misuse of Drugs Act 2001* and take into account the legal framework within which prescribing practice occurs. The scope of the policy includes developing a framework for the safe management of medicines, covering the handling and storage of medicines in accordance with the Duthie Report (Royal Pharmaceutical Society of Great Britain, 2005).

Non-medical prescribing forms part of the medicines management policy and should include details of the different roles and responsibilities of the prescriber, differentiating between independent prescribing, supplementary prescribing and PGDs. Included in the policy should be details of the requirements of the organisation and the non-medical prescriber in the correct issuing and security of prescription pads. There should be clear lines of accountability and a clear procedure to follow where security has been compromised or errors have occurred.

The recent reviews of mental health nursing in England and Scotland state that there needs to be the necessary governance in place before non-medical prescribing is developed (Snowden, 2007). This is in response to experiences of mental health practitioners who have undertaken training but then been unable to practise as a prescriber owing to systems and processes not being in place (National Prescribing Centre, 2005; Bradley et al., 2008).

Policies will also need to take into account future developments around electronic health records (Department of Health, 2001) and ensure that security of medicines and medicine prescribing is maintained.

Prescribing in mental heath

Prescribing in mental health may be perceived as an art. There are demands on clinicians to balance both pharmacological interventions with psychosocial interventions. There is also a huge demand when prescribing to address potential conflicts around achieving research/ evidence-based pharmacological interventions with practical considerations (e.g. costs) and the service user's wishes/desires (Jackson et al., 2003; Banning, 2004; National Prescribing Centre, 2007; Bradley et al., 2008).

All clinical interventions carry a risk potential. Ivan Illich (1976) referred many years ago to iatrogenesis and more recently we hear examples of significant numbers of service users – up to 10,000 in hospital settings – experiencing adverse reactions to medicines (Audit Commission, 2001). The National Patient Safety Agency (NPSA) provides a central point for reporting, monitoring and investigating adverse events (www.npsa.nhs.uk).

Any prescribing decisions require a risk–benefit analysis to ascertain a rationale for decisions that are made. This should be when initiating new treatments and when considering treatment changes (e.g. reduction/increases in dosages, switching from one medicine to another). The challenge for prescribers is to address appropriate prescribing practices with the hazards associated with medicines, including adverse reactions, side effects and interactions (Jackson et al., 2003; Bradley et al., 2007).

In a strategy to reduce risks, single medication (monotherapy) is often advocated as the simplest and safest route to prescribing (Doran, 2003). Wherever possible this should be utilised and is advocated by the National Institute for Clinical Excellence (NICE, www.nice.org.uk). Although there are clear benefits to monotherapy, in practice this can be immensely difficult as it fails to take into account existing co-morbidities (physical and mental ill health) and the value that some 'combination' therapies (polypharmacy) have in treating specific conditions (e.g. bipolar disorder, psychotic depression, etc.) as identified in prescribing guidelines (Taylor et al., 2007). There are, however, examples in the treatment of schizophrenia where up to 50% of service users are prescribed older (typical) and newer (atypical) antipsychotic medication at the same time (Harrington et al., 2002). This not only goes against NICE guidance but also significantly increases the risk factors associated with widening the side-effect profile of the medicines involved.

Seeking service users' views and involving carers and family as appropriate is key to engagement when making prescribing decisions and developing treatment plans. Developing a true concordant relationship is about having an appreciation of beliefs, understanding around illness and treatment, and working collaboratively to reach agreement on how treatment should proceed. Decisions on treatment, and particularly long-term treatment, should ideally take into account lifestyle factors. For example, if the service user is working they may not feel comfortable taking medication in the middle of their working day. Prescribing decisions would need to take account of this.

Regular reviews of medication are important in ensuring that drug treatment is being optimised with the risk of side effects being minimised. Reviews should consist of identifying requirements for good medicines management approaches, for example, when antipsychotics are prescribed, electrocardiogram (ECG), blood pressure (BP) and full blood count (FBC) should be monitored (Taylor et al., 2007) and use a recognised side-effect rating scale (National Prescribing Centre, 2005). Reviews should also take into account factors that are specific to the service user (substance misuse, co-morbidity, women of childbearing age, etc.), ensuring that safety is paramount in prescribing decisions.

The prescriber is accountable for ensuring that information concerning side effects, storage and disposal of the product is given to the service user/appropriate other. It is good practice to record in the notes that such information has been given (Nursing and Midwifery Council,

2005). Product licences also need to be considered. There are many occasions when medication is used outside of its product licence, for example drugs licensed for epilepsy used in mood stabilisation. However, the non-medical prescriber should only use unlicensed drugs when they are satisfied there is a good and cogent reason for it.

There has been criticism of the lack of appropriate interventions in mental health services to meet the physical health needs of mental health service users. Consequently, interventions to address physical care formed part of the Chief Nursing Officer's recommendations following a review of mental health nursing (Department of Health, 2006a). Caution is urged regarding the competence of mental health nurses to prescribe non-mental health drugs (National Prescribing Centre, 2005). Prescribing drugs for physical conditions may become part of the non-medical prescriber's scope of practice in mental health care, and steps to ensure the nurse can competently undertake this role is the responsibility of the employer and individual prescribing nurse.

Non-medical prescribers need to be aware of external influences on their prescribing choices as they may find themselves targeted by pharmaceutical representatives promoting their products (Davies & Hemingway, 2004). If the non-medical prescriber preferentially prescribes a product, he or she remains responsible for the appropriateness of the prescription, which should include checking the claims made for the product, and scrutinising the evidence base from studies on which the claims regarding the product are based. Evidence from NICE or guidance from the specialist psychiatric pharmacist are two sources that could be used. Box 4.10 summarises good prescribing practice.

Box 4.10 Summary of good prescribing practice

- Seek the service user's and carer's views on treatment.
- Adhere to local and national guidelines and protocols.
- Complete a risk–benefit analysis prior to prescribing decisions.
- Prescribe the least amount of medicines at the lowest possible doses.
- Discuss likely treatment outcomes and advise on possible side effects and interactions (including over-the-counter medicines).
- Regularly review, including monitoring of side effects using recognised rating scales.
- Consider service specific factors, e.g. co-morbidity, substance misuse and risk of pregnancy in women of childbearing age, etc.

Conclusions

This chapter has explored the establishment of frameworks and policies that need to be in place, and also the legal and professional issues that need to be considered for the non-medical prescriber to practise competently, safely and lawfully. There are factors external to the novice prescriber that are the responsibility of his or her employing authority, for example the establishment of clear and consistent policy so there is no confusion on the part of the prescriber. However, it is the individual prescriber's responsibility to understand policies and guidance from the law, work within them, and act reasonably in prescribing practice to promote beneficial psychopharmacological interventions, and minimise any likelihood of harm for the service user under his or her care.

We strongly recommend that you keep your knowledge of law up to date, as non-medical prescribing is an area of rapid expansion and change.

Acknowledgement

Special thanks to Barry Williams (Senior Lecturer) for his help and guidance and also to colleagues who have enabled us to cite examples from their clinical practice.

References

Audit Commission (2001) *Spoonful of Sugar*. Audit Commission, London.

Baird, A. (2004) Supplementary prescribing: one general practice's experience of implementation. *Nurse Prescribing*, **2**(2), 72–75.

Banning, M. (2004) Nurse prescribing, nurse education and related research in the United Kingdom: A review of the literature. *Nurse Education Today*, **24**, 420–427.

Bradley, E., Hynam, B. & Nolan, P. (2007) Nurse prescribing: reflections on safety in practice. *Social Science and Medicine*, **65**, 599–609.

Bradley, E., Wain, P. & Nolan, P. (2008) Putting mental health nurse prescribing in to practice. *Nurse Prescribing*, **6**(1), 15–19.

Caulfield, H. (1999) Nurse prescribing: a legal minefield? In: Jones, M. (ed.) *Nurse Prescribing: from Politics to Practice*. Bailliere Tindall, London.

Davies, J. & Hemingway, S. (2004) Pharmaceutical influences and nurse prescribers: eyes wide open? *Nurse Prescriber*, **1**(12), 224.

Department of Health (2000) *The NHS Plan: A Plan for Investment, a Plan for Reform*. Department of Health, London.

Department of Health (2001) *The Expert Patient – A New Approach to Chronic Disease Management for the 21st Century.* Stationary Office, London.

Department of Health. (2006a) *From Value to Actions: The Chief Nursing Officer's Review of Mental Health Nursing.* Department of Health, London.

Department of Health (2006b) *Improving Patients' Access to Medicines: A Guide to Implementing Nurse and Pharmacist Independent Prescribing.* Department of Health, London.

Department of Health (2007) *New Ways of Working for Everyone – A Best Practice Implementation Guide.* Department of Health, London.

Department of Health (2008) *Pharmacy in England: Building on Strengths – Delivering the Future.* Department of Health, London.

Dimond, B. (2008) *Legal Aspects of Mental Capacity.* Wiley-Blackwell, Oxford.

Doran, C. (2003) *Prescribing Mental Health Medication.* Routledge, London.

Fletcher, J. (2000) Some implications for nurses and managers of recent changes to the processing and hearing of medical negligence claims. *Journal of Nursing Management,* **8**(3), 133–140.

Foster, C. (2002) Negligence the legal perspective. In: Tingle, J. & Cribb, A. (eds) *Nursing Law and Ethics.* Blackwell Publishing, Oxford.

Gibson, B. (2001) Legal and accountability issues for nurse prescribing. In: Courtenay M. (ed.) *Current Issues in Nurse Prescribing.* Greenwich Media Ltd, London.

Harrington, M., Lelliott, P., Paton, C., Okocha, C., Duffett, R. & Sensky, T. (2002) The results of a multi-centre audit of the prescribing of antipsychotic drugs for in-patients in the UK. *Psychiatric Bulletin,* **26**, 414–418.

Hay, A. (2005) Examining the impact of non-medical prescribing in mental health. In: *South Staffordshire Healthcare NHS Trust.* Alton Towers, Staffordshire.

Hay, A., Bradley, E. & Nolan, P. (2004) Supplementary nurse prescribing. *Nursing Standard,* **18**(41), 33–39.

Healthcare Commission (2007) *Talking About Medicines. The Management of Medicines in Trusts Providing Mental Health Services.* Commission for Healthcare Audit and Inspection, London.

Hemingway, S. (2004) The mental health nurse's perspective on implementing nurse prescribing. *Nurse Prescribing,* **2**(1), 37–44.

Illich, I. (1976) *Limits to Medicine.* Penguin, London.

Jackson, S.H.D., Mangoni, A.A. & Batty, G.M. (2003) Optimization of drug prescribing. *British Journal of Clinical Pharmacology,* **57**(3), 231–236.

Joint Formulary Committee (2008) *British National Formulary.* British Medical Association and Royal Pharmaceutical Society of Great Britain, London.

Jones, A. (2008) Exploring independent prescribing for mental health settings. *Journal of Psychiatric and Mental Health Nursing,* **15**, 109–117.

Jones, M. & Jones, A. (2008) Choice as an intervention to promote well-being: The role of the nurse prescriber. *Journal of Psychiatric and Mental Health Nursing,* **15**, 75–81.

Jukes, M., Millard, J. & Chessum, C. (2004) Nurse prescribing: A case for clinical supervision. *British Journal of Community Nursing*, **9**(7), 291–297.

Kennedy, I. & Grubb, A. (2000) *Medical Law*. Butterworths, London.

Mazhindu, D. & Brownsell, M. (2003) Piecemeal policy may stop nurse prescribers fulfilling their potential. *British Journal of Community Nursing*, **8**(6), 253–255.

Medicines Act 1968 Available from www.statutelaw.gov.uk/content.aspx? LegType=All+Primary&PageNumber=62&NavFrom=2&parentActiveText DocId=1662209&activetextdocid=1662282 (accessed 01/07/08).

Mental Capacity Act 2005 Available from www.dca.gov.uk/menincap/ bill-summary.htm (accessed 30/07/08).

Mental Health Act 1983 Available from www.dh.gov.uk/en/Publicationsandstatistics/Legislation/Actsandbills/DH_4002034 (accessed 01/07/08).

Mental Health Amendments Act 2007 Available from www.opsi.gov.uk/acts/ acts2007/ukpga_20070012_en_1 (accessed 01/07/07).

Misuse of Drugs Act 2001 Available from www.opsi.gov.uk/si/si2001/20013998. htm (accessed 01/07/08).

Nash, M. (2005) Physical health care skills: A training needs analysis of inpatient and community mental health nurses. *Mental Health Practice*, **9**(4), 20–23.

National Prescribing Centre (2001) *A Competency Framework for Shared Decision Making with Patients*. National Prescribing Centre, Liverpool.

National Prescribing Centre (2005) *Improving Mental Health Services by Extending the Role of Nurses in Prescribing and Supplying Medication: Good Practice Guide*. NIMHE & NPC, London.

National Prescribing Centre (2007) *Maintaining Competency in Prescribing: An Outline Framework to Help Nurse Prescribers*. National Prescribing Centre, Liverpool.

Nolan, P. & Bradley, E. (2007) The role of the nurse prescriber: the views of mental health and non-mental health nurses. *Journal of Psychiatric and Mental Health Nursing*, **14**, 258–266.

Nursing and Midwifery Council (2004) *Guidelines for the Administration of Medicines*. Nursing and Midwifery Council, London.

Nursing Midwifery Council (2005) *Guidelines for Record and Record Keeping*. Nursing and Midwifery Council, London.

Nursing and Midwifery Council (2008) *Standards for Medicines Management*. Nursing and Midwifery Council London.

Otway, C. (2002) The development needs of nurse prescribers. *Nursing Standard*, **16**(18), 33–38.

Preece, S. (2002) Nurse prescribing: accountability and legal issues. In: Courtenay, M. & Butler, M. (eds) *Nurse Prescribing – Principles and Practice*. Oxford University Press, London.

Risk Review (2008) www.nps-riskconsulting.com.

Royal Pharmaceutical Society of Great Britain (2005) *The Safe and Secure Handling of Medicines: A Team Approach*. RPSGB, London.

Skingsley, D., Bradley, E. & Nolan, P. (2006) Neuropharmacology and mental health nurse prescribers. *Journal of Clinical Nursing*, **15**, 989–997.

Smith, M. & Hemingway, S. (2005) Developing as a nurse prescriber in mental health care: a case study. *Nurse Prescribing*, **3**(2), 79–84.

Snowden, A. (2007) Why mental health nurses should prescribe. *Nurse Prescribing*, **5**(5), 193–198.

Taylor, D., Paton, C. & Kerwin, R. (2007) *The Maudsley Prescribing Guidelines 2006–2007*. Taylor and Francis Group, London.

Weekes, L.M., Mackson, J.M., Fitzgerald, M. & Phillips, S.R. (2005) National Prescribing Service: creating an implementation arm for national medicines policy. *British Journal of Clinical Pharmacology*, **59**(1), 112–116.

While, A. & Biggs, K. (2004) Benefit and challenges of nurse prescribing. *Journal of Advanced Nursing*, **45**(6), 559–567.

Wix, S. (2007) Independent prescribing in the mental health setting. *Nursing Times*, **103**(44), 30–31.

Recovery and medication: a service user perspective

Michael Grierson

Introduction

I have worked in mental health services for over 20 years. I locate myself as part of the mental health user movement. There was only a short time – many moons ago – when I took psychiatric medication. The drugs were necessary and helpful for a while. Although I still believed myself to be Christ reborn, I felt a little less distressed and more in control of myself so I stopped taking all prescribed drugs. I thought that it was a sign of weakness to be taking psychiatric medication. I was wrong about that. I remember – and probably choose to remember – very little of this time in my life. However, I vividly recall being repeatedly told that I lacked insight into my condition and would come a cropper in due course. Good fortune, good friends and pursuit of a social science degree enabled me to get my life back on track.

In this chapter I want to have the discussion with the clinicians that was beyond me around 30 years ago. I want to express the anger, humiliation and lonely indignation that I felt being told that my only choice was the chemical restraint imposed upon me. Even at my craziest, there was much of me that understood the foolishness of my beliefs but I railed against being pilloried by medical personnel whom I saw as having their own delusions. The righteous wrath of Christ filled my mind – these people were beseeching me to rid myself of the troublesome speck in my eye, whilst oblivious to the plank in their own eyes. Moncrieff (2002) pinpointed the grievance that lay jumbled up inside me. She forcefully argued that psychiatric pharmacology is not even an inexact science; it is rather a non-science/a nonsense that has developed grandiose ideas of drugs influencing disease processes. The whole pretence of therapeutic practice hides the simple truth that psychiatric drugs are just sedating devices – no more, no less.

One very therapeutic tactic within the mental health user movement is table turning. This chapter will use this ploy outlining the fixed, false beliefs and lack of insight that leads clinicians to make poor decisions about psychiatric medication. I will describe the basics of what traditional clinicians do not know about psychiatric drugs and the people who are encouraged to take them for long periods of time. I will then chart the simple, practical advice that this service user critique proffers for practitioners to follow in their daily practice – the new deal that is being called for by the mental health user movement and progressive forces within mental health.

Lack of insight from traditional clinicians

With the readers' forbearance, I want to start by reminding you of a straightforward, if stereotypical, lived experience of being prescribed and taking psychiatric medication in the context of severe mental distress. I sense my non-existence, my inadequacy, my estrangement. In my desolate world, through glass, dimly I am aware of strange ideas fooling me and giving me pleasure. For a time I simply can not cope and I am in hospital. I think that I am Christ returned to painfully enable human nature to progress and reach a higher level of maturity. I guess that I presented as a classic schizophrenic – an emotional deadness combined with a lurid fantasy life. Not difficult to diagnose! The prognosis of doom that I was given both helped to confirm my own delusions and made me apoplectic (Deegan, 1988). I needed to take major tranquilisers and anti-psychotic medication for the next 70 years or so. The great revelations that I was experiencing were to be denied to the rest of the world as I became an enforced zombie. Different battles were raging in my head and one of them was a sensible me fighting the institutional manufacture of chronic mental illness as depicted by Estroff (1981).

Estroff (1981) sensitively observed the self-fulfilling prophecies of mental illness with which I was struggling. In terms of psychiatric medication, she identified the choice of symptoms that service users perceive. Whilst medicated people tend to be less thought disordered, they also tend to be more emotionally withdrawn, unable to experience any intensity of emotion. Many studies have related prolonged use of anti-psychotic medication to chronic apathy, depression, lack of energy and the dreaded onset of tardive dyskinesia (TD) (Hill, 1983). People are aware that there is a price to be paid for clinical improvement. The embarrassment, the feelings of dependence, the despair, and the restriction of activity have consequences not only in terms of self-image but in terms of people's ability to interact with others to whom medication and its so-called side effects are strange and stigmatising. Estroff (1981) argued that anti-psychotic drugs and major tranquilisers reduce the social expression of psychotic symptoms and contribute to personal and social disability. This was the choice that I dimly perceived at the time.

From time to time service users turn diagnostician. There may be money to be made in coming up with new disease classifications! Members of Survivors Speak Out (Lawson & Pembroke, 1994), for example, proposed a new entry for the *Diagnostic and Statistical Manual of Mental Disorders* (American Psychiatric Association, 1994). The main symptoms of professional thought disorder (PTD) are as follows.

Inappropriate affect
- Flat affect/cold professional demeanour.
- Marked social isolation within a certain professional group.
- Poverty of speech limited to brief conversations and avoidance of philosophical or ethical concerns.
- Marked lack of initiative and energy vis-à-vis getting to know about the patient's life.
- Absence of awareness or any sensitivity to spiritual experience, global feelings or ideas of transcendence.
- Rigidity of response in human relations.
- A general disregard for meaning in experience.
- Failure to notice or minimise any marked deficit in personality or functioning after another person's heavy drugging.

Bizarre delusions
- Delusion of biological reductionism – mental distress is caused by diseased cells/chemical imbalances.
- Delusion of non-connectedness of events – that events in the wider world have no meaningful connection to inner consciousness.
- Grandiose delusions – an exaggerated sense of one's self-importance, involving belief of professional expertise in, and ability to control, the innermost being of others.
- Belief in new drugs as panaceas.
- Compulsion to compartmentalise the experiences of others. In extreme cases this leads to complete de-personalisation.
- Rigidly held beliefs (called facts) that appear to be unaffected by empirical evidence from the real world.
- Tendency to ask strange questions which seem to have no relevance to context.

There is still too much PTD around today within services. I suffered from some of the iatrogenic effects of this condition. I felt patronised, ignored, hopeless, kept in the dark; I was made a passive recipient of treatment. When I was at a low ebb, I recall a consultant telling those around me that I was clearly much better. I have great empathy for the words of Deegan (2007):

'My psychiatrist said I was getting better, but I experienced being dis-abled by the medication. He said I was more in control, but I experienced the medication controlling me. He said my symptoms were gone, but my experience was that my symptoms were no longer bothersome to others but some continued to torment me. He said I had returned to baseline, but I experienced (not being myself anymore)'.

Deegan (2007), p. 63

It is a basic tenet of the mental health user movement that being on the receiving (rather than prescribing) end of psychiatric medication generally affords you a better understanding of the positive and nega-tive effects of treatment. Service user participants in a small, qualitative study by McGrath et al. (2007) make three key points about their expe-rience of psychiatric drugs. I have heard these points made many times over the years and I think they form a strong basis upon which to improve psychiatric medication practice.

One, psychosis needs drugs. Whatever the cause of psychotic break-down, there is not a lot that people can do when they are lost in the depths of fear and confusion. At this time people need becalming, to be reassured and cared for. When psychotic trauma passes, however, as it does for the vast majority of individuals, people need to be sup-ported to come off their medication or, at the very least, get by on minimum dosages. There needs to be a clear distinction between what is required during the acute phase of psychosis and the much longer period of rehabilitation and recovery.

Two, the long-term use of psychiatric medication often becomes an exercise in papering over the cracks. The root causes of distress in people's lives are ignored. In a world of risk management, it is argued that the consequence of suppressing underlying trauma by using drugs is as dangerous as suddenly not taking medication. Heavy medication regimes stop people from being able to deal with difficult realities and emotions in their lives. The whole enterprise becomes one of risk man-agement rather than recovery.

Three, drug-centred services rob people of their sense of self and their sense that they can actively do something to promote wellbeing in themselves. There is no human agency. One participant in the study makes the point succinctly:

'and then the next seventeen years, I was in and out of hospital 15 times, because I didn't know what to do to get well, even though as I said I had (a university education). I thought it was medication.'

McGrath et al. (2007), p. 6

The whole notion of recovery is about people being supported to find their own way out of the oppression of mental distress. In contradistinction to this approach, medication-based services can create dependencies and stigmatised identities. Clinical pessimism, low expectations, a paucity of rehabilitation support services and the relative security of welfare benefits are some of the aspects of the service system that encourage individuals to settle into mental illness careers. There is much that is comforting within illness and mental health care. Set against this, the idea of personal responsibility is a scary and thorny business, so it is little wonder than many opt for the patient role: I shall just take the drugs and trust to luck that I get better. There is nothing else that I can do. There are people who still live this philosophy. Too many people have been made passive by traditional psychiatry. The insistence upon compliance with drug regimes can relegate individuals to the role of passive patient; in effect, an object to be acted upon by mysterious experts.

Using psychiatric medication, rather than just taking it

Over many years I have asked service users what they do to improve their mental health – what their coping strategies are. No one has ever answered the question by mentioning psychiatric drugs. They take the drugs but do not think to mention them as part and parcel of their approach to developing better mental health. Many people, of course, do find psychiatric medication helps them. So why this omission? I feel it has to do with the compliance model that has hindered psychiatric practice for so long. The writings of a particularly articulate service user makes the argument. Pat Deegan (2007) pinpoints what many service users want as far as psychiatric drugs are concerned. People want choice, a sense of control and self-determination; they want their perspective and questions taken seriously and they want an honest dialogue with mental health practitioners.

Deegan (2007) developed the concept of personal medicine. It is a key notion here. It relates closely to the idea of a wellness toolbox, as expanded by Copeland (2008). Personal medicine comprises all the activities that you do to give your life meaning and purpose. On top of this, personal medicine consists of the self-care strategies that we each amass: all the things that we do to improve/stabilise our mood, suppress symptoms and generally lift or distract ourselves. For example, personal medicine can include going for walks in the countryside, exercise, spirituality, eating well, sex, shopping, sudoku, supporting a football team, being with friends, enjoying your own company, driving, pursuing a hobby or leisure pursuit, playing guitar, volunteering, reading, pottering about, etc. Importantly, personal medicine includes valued social roles that we have – parent, worker, friend and the like. Such roles give meaning, purpose and structure to what we do. They can motivate us to get up in the morning and do our best. They give us self-esteem. They can be a reason to carry on through hard times.

Just like 'pill' medicine, the self-care strategies and personal medicine that individuals find for themselves can be detrimental to health. For example, people use alcohol, illicit drugs and tobacco to self-medicate. Further, personal medication is not necessarily stress free as all social roles, valued or otherwise, involve elements of stress. Nonetheless, personal medicine is clearly vital to people's overall sense of wellbeing. Personal medicine is the strategy for living for each individual (Faulkner & Layzell, 2000). With this in mind, a huge problem that Deegan (2007) refers to is that many people do not disclose their personal medication regimes to their consultants. Moreover, when psychiatric drugs and their 'side effects' cause difficulties for personal medicine, this can lead people to discontinue their prescription and become non-compliant. For example, Roe and Swarbrick (2007) cite studies demonstrating a negative correlation between service users in employment and medication use. The suggestion here is that people in work will view medication in a poor light because of the associated stigma and problems with motivation.

In the old world view of non-compliance the expert clinician is depicted aside the recalcitrant, foolhardy service user. The latter, robbed of insight by delusions, stops taking medication and is soon overwhelmed by mental illness. All rationality is removed from this account. Best practice in medicine these days centres around the concept of concordance. Here, doctors and patients engage in a more human, cooperative and complex interaction. Through the consultation process, an agreement is reached about required medicine that respects the ideas and wishes of the patient. Heath (2003) argues that the concept of concordance masks the practical reality that patients' beliefs and needs are still paid scant attention.

Heath sees the notion of concordance as window dressing. Lip service is given to the principle that the patient's perspective is as valid as the clinician's. In truth, however, the principle that the 'doctor knows best' remains unquestioned. With concordance, Heath continues, the epistemological hierarchy (and concomitant treatment coercion) inherent within the compliance model remains but now it is concealed behind a veneer of respect. The patient is 'empowered' to comply through education and more information. Generally speaking, mainstream prescribing practice in psychiatry has a way to go in terms of genuinely respecting the self-determination of service users. A good starting point here would be more honest and better-informed dialogue about the uncertainties of psychiatric knowledge and the limitations of, and problems associated with, different psychiatric drugs. All patients need to be made aware of the pros and cons associated with drugs and then supported to make informed decisions.

This is just the approach that Deegan (2007) calls for. Individuals in need of psychiatric medication require a drug regime that works with their personal medicine and not against it. Deegan (2007) gives an example of a woman whose chief personal medicine was being a good mother. Psychotic depression hindered this principal role but so did her prescribed medication so she stopped taking it. After a period of being non-compliant, the woman worked with a nurse prescriber and together they found a medication regime that enhanced her personal medicine. They painstakingly found a way to reduce symptoms without zombifying her so that she was able to take care of her children. In this case, the credit for improved clinical and social outcomes can be attributed to both psychiatric medication and the woman's determination to be there for her kids.

On a daily basis I see people who attribute any and all improvement in their wellbeing to the medication that they have been on for so many years. I feel that so much is frequently missed from this account. As Deegan (2005) states:

> 'recovery is hard work and it requires personal agency, will, vision, hope, fortitude, courage, imagination, commitment, and resilience.'

> Deegan (2005), p. 34

The beauty of the concept of personal medicine is that it enables people to see their role in their recovery journey. Never again should all of the credit go to pharmaceuticals. The medical model that has promulgated this is incredibly disempowering and it is wildly simplistic. All mental health service users need to be removed from the straitjacket of their allotted role as outpatients faithfully taking pills. People need to be supported to actively use their medication to bolster their personal strengths in pursuit of a better life.

Towards making better decisions about psychiatric medication

From a service user perspective, the problematic issue of non-compliance is not so much to do with individuals wrongly believing that they have no need for medication because they are not really ill. Rather, it has more to do with a difficult personal choice focused upon pursuing activities that give life meaning and value. Many people continue to make unwise decisions about coming off medications. Others make unwise decisions to stay being over-medicated for fear of the consequences. One of the difficulties with psychiatric medication is that it can be an absolutist arena. You are for them or against them. Some service users want to stay with their prescribed medication regime at all costs. Others want to get off their psychiatric drugs at all costs. Some people are too frightened to look at the risks associated with their treatment. Others only see the risks.

As recovery principles imbibe psychiatric medication practice, the cultural shift is towards service users and clinicians working together to devise an ongoing and mutually acceptable plan aimed at using drugs alongside other coping strategies to manage symptoms and get on with life. The task is to get both prescriber and outpatient to assume responsibilities in this process. In addition, the task is to build trust and respect between mental health professionals and service users. This involves practitioners learning to listen to service users and genuinely appreciate what they are saying, even and especially when clinician and client disagree. We need to do better than the traditional model of non-compliance. In this model the doctor feels satisfied because symptoms have abated. The patient is depressed because they sense that the price that they are paying is a social disability and alienation from their real self. They feel drugged up to the eyeballs. There is no meaningful communication in this 'therapeutic' encounter and the patient quietly stops taking their medication.

Both clinician and service user can do better than this. My reading of recovery-oriented literature and my personal and work experience lead me to proffer this simple advice for both service users and service providers as they face their decision-making responsibilities. As for mental health professionals and the service system: It needs to be the central tenet of all future services that by far the most therapeutic element of psychiatric care is not any treatment on offer but the quality of the working relationship that is developed between mental health professional and service user (Repper & Perkins, 2003). Services and structures need to be devised that honour and apply this principle. For example, Hall (2007) rightly points out that the typical outpatient consultation does not provide the time and context for the proper discussion of mental health and medication issues. There are examples of how services can be better structured to foster hope-inspiring professional practice developing all the time (Abrahamson, 1991). Professional training programmes should focus upon the minutia of developing a trusting rapport with service users, rather than relationship skills being the great taken-for-granted within clinical education.

A key aspect of professional practice that will promote trusting relationships is the sharing of information and the answering of people's questions. Individuals have damn good questions concerning their medication. What are these drugs doing to my liver/sex life/my motivation? Have my medication needs not changed over the past 10 years because I have been on exactly the same medication over this time? What are the risks with long-term use of this medication? In my role as advocate I have supported many people to attend outpatient consultation meetings where they have gone to have questions answered. Far too many times their questions have been ignored and treated as insignificant or silly. Time and again I have witnessed consultants respond to good questions by laughing or smiling inappropriately (much as Dr Hibbert does in The Simpsons), and then proffering unrelated advice. Such advice has included 'You need to leave the parental home and get away from your mother's apron strings', 'Get yourself a girlfriend', 'You need to chill out and have a few beers', and 'You need to get into the garden and build yourself a shed'! Truth be told, we could have gone to the pub and the guy next to us at the bar would have given us the same advice. It is bar-room banter, not professional practice. The space, time and rationale for discussing the benefits, drawbacks and risks of taking specific drugs needs to be built in. There is, of course, a wealth of information on the physical and mental health effects of taking psychiatric medication.

Medication needs to be discussed as one coping tool amongst many. Furthermore, for choice to become a meaningful notion within services, there needs to be the option of professional support to come off medications as greater reliance upon other coping strategies is fostered. Practitioners need to find out about and support people's personal medicine strategies. The current cultural shift is from engendering a passive hope in the magic of psychiatric drugs to enabling people to take an active role amidst the challenges they face. Medication management needs to take its place within this zeitgeist. Clinicians must painstakingly explore with service users how pill medicine supports personal medicine in an ongoing journey. Clinicians need to familiarise themselves with, and build upon, the fantastic coping strategies that service users have developed for themselves and the breathtaking resilience that they demonstrate in dealing with difficulties (Faulkner & Layzell, 2000).

There does need to be far better practice vis-à-vis research in the whole field of psychiatric medication. Better practice will range from more focused research into how effective drugs are in leading to improved outcomes in people's lives to more investigation of the lived experience of people who have successfully withdrawn from psychiatric medication. It (almost) goes without saying that the menacing power of drug companies needs to be counterbalanced by commissioners of future evidence-based services.

There needs to be a greater focus on the structure of practise around medication issues, for example exploring the distinction between short-term and long-term use of drugs. In their recommendations for practice, McGrath et al. (2007) empathise that the service user perspective clearly differentiates between using medication in usually short-lived acute, psychotic periods and the use of medication in the longer haul of a recovery journey. To the extent that current service provision is obsessed by risk management rather than recovery, there needs to be good risk assessment of keeping people on high dosages of medication for longer than is required.

The development of better practice in the prescribing, monitoring and evaluation of medication necessitates that service users and user-led services take up more responsibilities. Key duties include:

- Individual service users need to share their personal medicine strategies with their clinicians. Treatment options need to be discussed in relation to personal goals, social roles and our private coping strategies. Service users themselves need to appreciate just how important and effective their personal coping strategies and resilience are. People who have learnt to stigmatise themselves need to relearn to trust themselves and not give all the credit to a set of chemicals.
- User-led services and peer support structures need to provide more support to enable individuals to learn from others about exactly how psychiatric drugs have helped them in the recovery journey. Roe & Swarbrick (2007) encourage nurses to teach service users about how some people have learnt to cope with 'side effects' of drugs. There is plenty of scope for user-led groups and mental health professionals to work together in educating staff and service users about developing positive practice in medication.
- Service users need to learn to speak assertively with consultants, rather than passively or aggressively. If clinician and service user are to work collaboratively, service users must learn to think differently about medication, think differently about themselves and think differently about consultants (Deegan, 2005, 2007). Service users need to be supported to actively take their role in this working relationship – to believe that their questions are important and to see the strengths and limitations to psychiatric expertise. Strong peer support is a must to prepare service users for their 'work' with clinicians and fight learned helplessness. User-led services need to be better resourced to make this peer support a reality.

Deegan (2007) talks about the skill building required of service users as they train to use psychiatric drugs as one tool in their recovery journey. Skills include techniques to distract your attention from distressing symptoms, finding ways to exercise which produces many physical and emotional benefits, learning ways to quieten your thoughts – in short, the whole myriad of self-care and coping strategies. Again, peer support structures are an ideal setting for sharing and exploring the developing database of options in strategies for living. The report by Faulkner & Layzell (2000) is a fine starting point for groups to look at the strengths and limitations of their own coping strategies and peer support groups can empower people to practise coping skills.

One required option amongst peer support groups is user-led medication reduction support groups. Psychiatric drugs are extremely useful at different times in people's lives. Some of the short-term benefits, such as getting some sleep when your mind is out of control, are life savers. Hall (2007) outlines some of the many ways in which people benefit from their medication – in the short-term. People can only exercise meaningful choice if mental health services make drug-free psychiatric care a genuine option. For this to be the case, again, peer support needs to be resourced and service users need to work collaboratively with practitioners such as the community pharmacy service and nurses in the running of groups to discuss medication in a thorough and balanced manner.

There; I have finished my long-overdue rant. What is the point of psychiatric medication? To help people on their recovery journey. The developing therapeutic alliance asks a lot from clinicians. Practitioners need to balance optimism and realism, treat service users as equals, believe in people when they do not believe in themselves and support people to accept and learn from setbacks as part of the recovery process. Medication management takes its place within this context.

References

Abrahamson, D. (1991) A combined group and individual long-term out-patient clinic. *Psychiatric Bulletin*, **15**, 486–487.

American Psychiatric Association (1994) *Diagnostic and Statistical Manual of Mental Disorders*, 4th edn. American Psychiatric Association, Washington DC.

Copeland, M.E. (2008) www.mentalhealthrecovery.com/.

Deegan, P.E. (1988) Recovery: The lived experience of rehabilitation. *Psychosocial Rehabilitation Journal*, **9**(4), 11–19.

Deegan, P.E. (2005) The importance of personal medicine: A qualitative study of resilience in people with psychiatric disabilities. *Scandinavian Journal of Public Health*, **33**(Suppl 66), 29–35.

Deegan, P.E. (2007) The lived experience of using psychiatric medication in the recovery process and a shared decision-making program to support it. *Psychiatric Rehabilitation Journal*, **31**(1), 62–69.

Estroff, S. (1981) *Making It Crazy*. University of California Press, California.

Faulkner, A. & Layzell, S. (2000) *Strategies for Living: A Report of User-Led Research into People's Strategies for Living with Mental Distress*. The Mental Health Foundation, London.

Hall, W. (2007) *Harm Reduction Guide to Coming Off Psychiatric Drugs*. The Icarus Project and Freedom Center, New York.

Heath, I. (2003) A wolf in sheep's clothing: a critical look at the ethics of drug taking. *British Medical Journal*, **327**, 856–858.

Hill, D. (1983) *The Politics of Schizophrenia*. University Press of America, London.

Lawson, D. & Pembroke, L. (1994) Professional Thought Disorder. *Asylum*.

McGrath, P., Bouwman, M. & Kalyanasundaram, V. (2007) 'A very individual thing': Findings on drug therapy in psychiatry from the perspective of Australian consumers. *Australian e-Journal for the Advancement of Mental Health*, **6**(3), 1–11.

Moncrieff, J. (2002) Drug treatment in modern psychiatry: the history of a delusion. In: Critical Psychiatry Network (ed.) *Beyond Drugs and Custody: Renewing Mental Health Practice*. Paragon Hotel, Birmingham.

Repper, J. & Perkins, R. (2003) *Social Inclusion and Recovery. A Model for Mental Health Practice*. Balliere Tindall, London.

Roe, D. & Swarbrick, M. (2007) A recovery-oriented approach to psychiatric medication: guidelines for nurses. *Journal of Psychosocial Nursing and Mental Health Services*, **45**(2), 35–40.

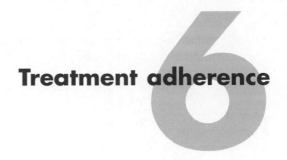

Treatment adherence

Neil Harris

Introduction

Prescribing a medication regimen that service users are willing and able to take is a major concern for mental health practitioners. Adherence is a complex phenomenon, with many variables associated with it being unique to the individual, his or her circumstances and the care team. It is often surrounded with complicated and paradoxical clinical and ethical dilemmas and causes strong emotions in the service user, family and care team. This chapter aims to explore some of the key issues in treatment adherence and offers good practice points for work in this area.

What are we talking about – compliance, adherence, concordance?

One of the first attempts to define the concept was made by Haynes in 1976:

> 'The extent to which a person's behaviour (taking medications, following a recommended diet, or executing life-style changes) coincides with the medical advice given.'

More recently the term 'adherence' has become preferable as it is thought to put a greater emphasis on the development of a therapeutic alliance. This enables the active participation of the service user in the process of medicines management. But when does non-adherence occur? Is it when service users adjust their regimen to suit themselves, only taking medication when feeling stressed, or is it only when they decide to stop taking their prescribed medication?

Concordance is a conceptualisation of the relationship between the service user and the prescriber. It describes a negotiated agreement between the service user and a healthcare professional that determines whether, when and how medicines are to be taken. It embodies the notion of an alliance, where practitioners recognise the authority the service user has in medication decision-making. The result of this negotiation would be a prescription the person agrees to take and in this sense embodies the essence of informed consent.

However, this process may leave the care team with emotional, ethical and legal conflicts when trying to marry the practice of evidence-based care with a service user's preference, such as only taking a sub-optimal dose of medication (Merinker & Shaw, 2003). This work is managing these conflicts, developing low-risk strategies and supporting people to make decisions and learn from their experience.

How widespread is non-adherence to medication in mental health?

Adherence is not just an issue that is confined to mental health services. In most medical conditions the rates of non-adherence are high: 40% in the treatment for tuberculosis, approaching 50% for antibiotics and nearly 40% of people prescribed cardiovascular medication are considered non-adherent (Ley & Llewellyn, 1995). For mental health conditions the adherence rates are variable; for people prescribed antidepressants non-adherence is estimated at between 30 and 60% (Demyttenaere, 1998). For schizophrenia it has been estimated that around 50% of service users do not take their medication regimen (Fenton et al., 1997; Lacro et al., 2002) and further studies indicate that between 30 and 50% adjust the dose of their medication (Hornung et al., 1998; Verdoux et al., 2000). In bi-polar disorders between 20 and 66% of service users do not adhere to their treatment (Lingam et al., 2002).

The wide range of estimates given for adherence to treatment indicates the difficulties presented in this area of enquiry. There are a number of factors which contribute to the methodological problems in conducting research of this nature – the study design, the definition given to the 'medication taking behaviour', the method used to measure non-adherence, the number of service users evaluated – and it may be that the people who decide not to adhere to treatment may also be unwilling to take part in the research exploring this behaviour, making the research unrepresentative. Nevertheless, experts have concluded that poor adherence is a common problem in mental health, having a major impact on the effectiveness of therapeutic interventions and on the clinical management of conditions.

Factors affecting adherence

The causes of non-adherence to treatment are wide ranging and are often interconnected and complex. Several factors have been identified which increase or decrease the likelihood that a person will follow treatment prescriptions, and are commonly categorised into four groups (Fenton et al., 1997; Oehl et al., 2000):

- *Patient-related factors*: socio-demographic variables including age, gender, social status, educational level, the type, phase and severity of illness, and specific symptoms such as paranoia, grandiosity, delusional beliefs, depression, cognitive impairment and negative symptoms. Awareness of illness, insight and the need for treatment as well as a person's health beliefs and beliefs about medicines in general are implicated in taking medication.
- *Environmental factors*: including the views and opinions of relatives and friends, and their willingness and/or availability to support and assist or supervise medication. Local arrangements for collection of medication and environmental cues and prompts to take the medication can also be a factor.
- *Clinician-related factors*: an open and genuine therapeutic alliance with members of the care team and the service user's perception of the practitioner's interest in him or her as a person was found to be a strong predictor of medication adherence (Lindstrom et al., 2000), as was lack of coercion and increased involvement in decision-making (Day et al., 2005).
- *Treatment-related factors*: factors which increase the likelihood of non-adherence include complex treatment regimens, the presence and/or severity of side effects and the perceived effectiveness of therapy. Adherence may also be altered according to the label, package or form of the medication, and also by the type and financial consideration if the person is paying for his or her prescription.

Issues in clinical practice

Effective medicines management work is grounded in the relationship between the practitioner and service user. The quality of the relationship between members of the care team and service user is not only influential in the person's decision to take medication in the first place but also in facilitating meaningful discussions about self-efficacy and management as treatment progresses. The level of the practitioner's knowledge, regarding pharmacology and medicines management, has an impact on their stance towards treatment (Bryne et al.,

2005). Higher levels of understanding facilitate more positive attitudes towards medication and working with people in this area. This emphasises the key role practitioners play in helping people to get the most from medication.

In inpatient settings, the therapeutic alliance with practitioners, lack of coercion and involvement in treatment decisions are important factors in encouraging adherence (Day et al., 2005). Encouraging an atmosphere for open and frank discussions can help the person develop greater understanding of medication issues and the complexities of management. These discussions can set the conditions for people to make positive decisions about how they can use medication in recovery (National Institute for Mental Health England, 2005). In this context, working in partnership with users and carers develops an awareness regarding the need to offer treatment alternatives, if medication side effects compromise their ability to achieve vocational and social goals.

This relationship may not be easy to establish or sustain and many situations can undermine the positive understanding that has developed. Poor experience with treatment, symptoms, insight and chaotic lifestyles and entrenched, inflexible and paternalistic professional attitudes are some of the problems associated with difficulties in establishing and maintaining a rapport. The emotional concern practitioners can feel for people who choose to discontinue medication or only agree with sub-optimal doses can result in over-assertive strategies in an attempt to avoid a relapse. Finding themselves in this situation the service user may decide that the only way to avoid confrontation is by covert action. Awareness of such a circumstance, developing and addressing the issue, can avoid the breakdown of the relationship. In clinical practice it is far better to work in a way where the person feels they can be open and honest, able to say they have decided to discontinue their medication, than be kept in the dark because they were too afraid to let it be known. Openness in this area can enable decisions to be supported and the integrity of partnership working maintained, facilitating future action if needed.

Practitioners must always act in the best interest of the service user (Nursing and Midwifery Council, 2004). This can cause difficulties within the multi-disciplinary team as conflicting views can be voiced regarding what is in the best interest of the service user regarding medication decisions. An aspect of the practitioner's role is to ensure that the service user's views are heard, along with information that has informed this view. Sometimes it is difficult to advocate in this way, especially when it contradicts the views of other, perhaps more experienced, practitioners.

It may frequently be the case that when undertaking medicines management work, the relationship with the service user and carers, and/or professional relationships with colleagues, can be compromised when difficult circumstances and complex clinical situations arise. At these times the management of conflicts with interpersonal skills, and an awareness of the diverse values which may be influencing behaviour and communication, can form the focus of work that needs resolution. Woodbridge & Fulford (2004) suggest a three-phase strategy to improving communication when interpersonal conflicts occur between service users, carers or other practitioners.

The first stage is a reflective process which seeks to develop an individual's awareness of the content of the communication and their contribution to the dynamics within the exchange:

- the attitude they have towards the person and the stance they are projecting towards them;
- what is getting in the way of listening to what the person has to say and how is the other person perceiving their willingness to listen and understand;
- what information is the person communicating;
- the level of self-awareness of the practitioners' mental processes whilst listening to the person.

The second stage is concerned with the skills and attitudes the person needs in order to move through the conflict towards resolution:

- acknowledging that different perspectives are part of everyday life and are valuable;
- an empathic stance which shows a willingness to accept the person and work with the person to understand his or her point of view.

The third stage addresses the information the person is communicating without trying to discredit his or her position and prove him or her wrong:

- maintain a reflective outlook, observing for personal barriers to effective communication.

Enabling service users to become effective partners in their health care

A structure of good practice for developing a dialogue with a service user to reach agreement regarding treatment can be found in *A Competency Framework for Shared Decision-making with Patients* (National Prescribing Centre, 2007). The project worked from the position that 'shared decision-making' and 'medicines concordance' are interchangeable; the common focus of a partnership in care enabling service users to make informed decisions about their treatment. The framework was developed as a template to assist all healthcare practitioners to engage in effective consultations with service users. The framework has been adjusted to take account of working with people with mental health problems. It should also be noted that making decisions about a person's treatment often involves other people: carers, other family members, and sometimes friends or advocates. The structure provided here can be used when discussing medication with them.

The framework is constructed on three levels:

1. *Building a partnership.* This provides details of the components of developing a therapeutic relationship with the person. This includes:
   - demonstrating understanding through the use of summaries, showing sensitivity and empathy, and valuing the person's viewpoint
   - using interpersonal skills by being open and answering questions, communicating in a style which is non-critical and shows warmth, concern and caring
   - collaborating; offering choices, encouraging and accepting suggestions, seeking positive and negative feedback.
2. *Managing a shared consultation.* This involves developing an agenda and rationale for the meeting, enabling a discussion that is clear in focus and boundaries, and seeks to gain an understanding regarding the service users' desired level of involvement in their treatment decisions. As in all areas of health care, practitioners are expected to maintain up-to-date knowledge, develop skills, know their limitations and when to get advice or make a referral. The framework emphasises working closely with other practitioners, sharing information about specialist support, and community and practical resources.
3. *Sharing a decision.* This third level of the framework is divided into four domains. They do not operate in a sequential way but interact in the consultation:
   - Understanding: involves getting to know the person, their culture and living arrangements, family and friends, asking questions to find out about their current situation and experience of mental health problems and services. Exploring cultural, religious and health beliefs and those beliefs that may be connected with their mental health problem will help develop an awareness of aspects that affects their position to medication. Finding out about their supports, resources and assets is important information when agreeing plans and care. It is important to respect, acknowledge and use the person's expertise of their own condition and

treatment experiences in setting goals. It is also important to discuss their readiness to take a decision and make a change, as it is their views that will dictate what to do next.

- *Exploring*: aims to find out about the person's mental health problems and develop treatment options. Questions are used to explore the person's understanding of their illness, what they think about their symptoms, why they occur and how they are best managed. Guided discovery can be used to examine what strategies and techniques the person uses to cope with symptoms, how effective they are and whether improvements can be made. This technique can also develop detail regarding other aspects of their mental health problems and medicines management issues. Enquiries should be made about their views on medicines in general, perhaps using the health beliefs model as a guide to discussion. Similarly, discussion about their treatment may reveal expectations and concerns that require action to be taken or the provision of information. The provision of information about the person's mental health problems is an essential part of this dialogue and may result in a difference of opinion between the practitioner and service user regarding illness and symptoms. It is important to address these differences in a way which is not challenging or threatening but enables the person to explore different experiences and meanings, including their positive and negative views about treatment and the option of no treatment at all.

- *Deciding*: requires working through a number of treatment issues with the person in order to agree a medication strategy. The provision of full and accurate information about the pros and cons of all treatment options is an essential component in enabling the person to make an informed decision. As part of this discussion the practitioner should give information about the course of illness and possible treatment outcomes, including areas of risk and uncertainty. In the context of providing the service user with sufficient information on which to base a decision, it is important for practitioners to explain their stance regarding medication and provide a rationale for its use or why it may not be necessary. Based on this information the practitioner and service user can negotiate a treatment decision, and check whether the person understands the reasons behind the decision. After service users have had time to consider their chosen option the practitioner needs to accept this decision, clarifying with the service users the details about the agreed treatment plan and their rationale for agreement. Finally, detail can be sought regarding the person's ability to carry out the agreed plan, anticipating problems which might occur and, if necessary, problem solving to identify solutions.

■ *Monitoring*: is the final domain and is an integral part of medicines management. It is the means by which medication changes are indicated and provides a prompt for a speedy response. Establishing a course of action should problems occur, a relapse prevention plan, is good practice. Monitoring is also about identifying positive symptom changes, or reduced or eliminated side effects that can lead to dosage changes, reducing risk and increasing the potential for further benefit, and this information should be sought. A review can bring this information together to guide future decisions. Details regarding a review date and the readiness to review the decision should be established.

The framework gives clear guidance on the competencies required (knowledge, skills and attitudes) to undertake effective discussions with service users, which will enable them to take an active part in sharing the treatment decisions.

Assessment and intervention

As stated earlier, the beliefs the person has regarding medication is one of the factors that influence adherence. The development of the health belief model (Rosenstock, 1975) has enhanced the understanding of the decision-making process people use when making choices regarding health care. The model asserts that people make rational decisions based on their judgement as to whether the benefits of a suggested course of treatment outweigh the disadvantages. For people with psychotic disorders this position is sometimes compromised by lack of insight, where the person does not appreciate the costs involved in non-adherence, or cognitive impairments, like poor memory, concentration or attention, resulting in lack of understanding regarding the benefits of treatment (Corrigan, 2002).

The Brief Evaluation of Medication Influences and Beliefs (BEMIB) scale is a short, validated eight-item assessment of adherence to treatment based on the treatment expectancies described in the health beliefs model (Dolder et al., 2004) (Figure 6.1). Developed from earlier work by Perkins (1999, 2002) the eight statements in the scale refer to five domains:

- benefits of treatment, in terms of symptom control and hospitalization;
- risks of becoming ill, regarding being insightful into the need for medication;

- costs of treatment, in terms of side-effect experience and difficulties in obtaining the medication;
- obstacles to adherence, referring to administration and support issues;
- prompts to ensure administration, referring to the use of medication management strategies.

In this scale higher scores indicate positive attitudes and beliefs towards medication, whereas low scores are associated with non-adherence. The scale is useful as it can be undertaken and analysed quickly and, although presented here as a measure for exploring the use of antipsychotic medications, the wording can be changed to facilitate its use with other medications and service user groups. Information gained as a result of conducting the assessment can be used to develop care plans and target interventions to address the barriers to adherence. The issue of providing information will be discussed at the end of the section as it provides the foundation of much of valuable work that can be undertaken as part of medicines management. The statements in the scale will now be looked at individually to explore the issues in each domain and the interventions and stance taken to address problematic areas.

1. Taking my medication makes me feel better

People should feel a benefit from taking a medication but for many psychotropic medications there is a variation in response. Antipsychotic medication, when used to treat psychosis, is ineffective for between 5 and 25% of people prescribed it (Conley & Buchanan, 1997). Ensuring that the service user is prescribed the most effective regimen can be a difficult and lengthy business. Maintaining an accurate medication history can be a key factor in enabling changes that may be more beneficial. Regular assessment and monitoring of symptoms can help the service user to make informed judgements about efficacy, especially when tracked against previous assessments and drug regimens. Discussions between the service user and family members where appropriate, and the care team can refine the prescription. The 'pros and cons' exercise, described in Chapter 12 is a useful way of helping service users to evaluate and appraise their medication experience.

2. Taking my medication helps prevent me getting hospitalized

The changing role of medication over the course of a person's illness is not always clearly explained to the service user. Initial prescriptions to eliminate acute, distressing symptoms can change to maintenance

My antipsychotic medication(s)...

The following questions involve your antipsychotic medication. There are no right or wrong answers, but your honest response is important. Please respond to the following statements regarding your medication by circling the answer that best matches how you agree or disagree.

	Completely disagree	Generally disagree	Undecided (neither agree or disagree)	Generally agree	Completely agree
1.Taking my antipsychotic medication makes me feel better	1	2	3	4	5
2. Taking my antipsychotic medication helps to prevent me getting hospitalized	1	2	3	4	5
3. Side effects from my antipsychotic medication bother me	5	4	3	2	1
4. I have a system (e.g. pill-box, medication calendar, someone giving me my antipsychotic medication) that helps me remember to take my antipsychotic medication	1	2	3	4	5
5. Taking my antipsychotic medication is difficult to remember everyday	5	4	3	2	1
6. Getting my medication from the hospital or pharmacy is not a problem	1	2	3	4	5
7. I am supported by my family, friends and doctor to take my medication	1	2	3	4	5
8. I have a psychiatric disorder that antipsychotic medication improves	1	2	3	4	5

Figure 6.1 The Brief Evaluation of Medication Influences and Beliefs scale (Dolder et al., 2004).

or relapse prevention treatment once symptoms in the acute phase have diminished. Without information regarding this change of use, service users may discontinue medications when they become free of distressing experiences. Titrating doses downwards to enable relapse prevention at the lowest possible dose is a difficult process. For example, if a service user is symptom-free, under-dosing can occur which can result in a deteriorating mental state and relapse. Similarly a low-dose regimen may enable service users to remain well over a long period of time, maintaining them in their stress-vulnerability threshold, until a significant life event exposes them to increased stress, increasing their vulnerability to experiencing symptoms. Enabling the person to receive the lowest dose of a medication needed to remain well is a principle of good practice in the pharmacological treatment of long-term mental illness; however, the process of establishing and maintaining this regimen is not without risk. Service users, carers and care staff need to be mindful of these risk factors and have agreement for undertaking early warning signs work and developing an action plan. Helping the service user to establish a link between medication adherence and periods of illness and distress is a valuable therapeutic intervention that can be aided with the use of a time line (see Chapter 11 for an explanation of this technique).

3. Side effects from my medication bother me

For some people the experience of side effects of medication can be mild and transitory while others can develop effects that can be persistent and/or severe. Furthermore the 'cost' a service user is willing to tolerate when balanced against symptom relief is variable. Side effects are often cited as reasons why a service user takes the decision to discontinue a medication, preferring symptoms to adverse drug effects. Systematic and regular assessment of the side effects should form a fundamental role in managing a person's health care although this does not always happen in clinical practice (see Chapter 10).

There are a number of strategies aimed at reducing side-effect experience. One often suggested strategy involves switching the person's prescription to a similar medication from a different chemical group. However, this does not always work. For example, in the case of antipsychotics it is often stated that atypical medications provide an improved side-effect profile and are therefore better tolerated by service users, increasing adherence. However, recent research has suggested that significant numbers of service users discontinue medication, irrespective of whether they are prescribed atypical or conventional preparations, due to lack of efficacy, side effects or other reasons (Lieberman et al., 2005).

4. I have a system (e.g. pill-box, medication calendar, someone giving me my antipsychotic medication) that helps me remember to take my antipsychotic medication

Behavioural tailoring involves working with service users to fit taking medication into their daily routine. Tailoring the administration of medication to a recurring daily event, like taking with the evening meal or putting medication next to the toothbrush to prompt administration before brushing, has shown to be effective for some people (Mueser et al., 2002). The use of a dosette box, a container compartmentalised to fit administration times, has been shown to aid adherence and can be filled on a weekly basis by the service user or family member. Medication can often be dispensed in this form by local chemists. Some people may find a telephone prompt useful either as an initial aid to getting into a routine or on a more long-term basis. This kind of assistance can often be negotiated with the care team.

5. Taking my antipsychotic medication is difficult to remember everyday

Unintentional partial or total non-adherence to medication is one aspect in the area of adherence. Difficulties can arise for a service user who has accepted the need for medication but does not take the prescription. In this situation practitioners can assume that persistent symptoms or a slow deterioration in mental state is a result of poor response to treatment, rather than under-dosing, and can result in increases in dosage, change to another preparation or polypharmacy. As discussed earlier, many people forget to take a prescribed medication or a course of antibiotics, for example. For a range of mental health problems this position is further hampered by cognitive deficits, experienced as part of the condition itself or as side effects of the medication. These difficulties not only result in problems in providing and retaining information generally but also increase problems with understanding and remembering instructions for administration. In terms of adherence there is a benefit to be gained in simplifying the regimen and tailoring administration to the individual's circumstances.

Finding out the service user's preference for drug formulation is an important part of the medication management decision-making process, and for service users and practitioners conventional oral preparations, tablets and capsules are the stated preference (Müller, 2006). Although some people may prefer the treatment delivered in long-acting depot form, to avoid the daily process of administration, this treatment option must be based on the person's decision.

Simplifying the drug regimen can increase the probability that the person will take the medication. Reducing the number of different types of drugs a person is prescribed is a key factor in this process and not only makes administration much more straightforward and reduces the risk of administration error but confers a number of other advantages. It reduces the range of dangerous complications, side effects and potential for drug interactions associated with multiple prescriptions, and also enables the service user and care team to monitor the effectiveness of the treatment. In this context the regimen can be examined to find ways of discontinuing unnecessary prescriptions, for example dose reduction instead of routine prescription of anticholinergic preparations or switching to clozapine instead of polypharmacy with multiple antipsychotics. However, this process is complicated by the benefits sometimes conferred by the use of adjunctive medications for the treatment of multiple symptom experiences. An additional complication in this area is when a service user is receiving input from a number of medical services, the general practitioner (GP), psychiatrist and general specialists. Contact with multiple services can result in overly complicated regimens, with increased risk of contra-indications and interactions.

An aim of prescription would be to establish the service user on a single daily dose of medication. Evidence has suggested that adherence decreases as the number of times the person is expected to take medication in a day increases – 'Take this tablet once a day' is more likely to be followed than 'Take these three tablets four times a day'. Targeting the use of antipsychotics that only require a single daily dose, such as olanzapine, aripirazole or risperidone, may be a factor to consider when negotiating treatment decisions (Burton, 2005).

Problem solving is a skill that is used for addressing these and other problematic areas. Becoming proficient at these skills is useful, not only for issues related to medicines management but for many aspects of the person's life. The intervention of such a crucial aspect of medicines management is looked at in greater detail in Chapter 12.

6. Getting my medication from the hospital or pharmacy is not a problem

Organising the most convenient arrangements for service users to collect their medication is an important aspect of sorting out the practical issues of medication management. The choice of where to collect medication from may not solely depend on access to the nearest chemist but can include other considerations such as the service of dispensing of medication in dosette boxes. It may be more convenient for the service user to cash his or her prescription at the hospital pharmacy following an outpatient appointment or during a meeting with a member of the care team. It has been proposed that prescription charges have resulted in non-redemption of prescriptions and thus provides a further dimension to non-adherence. Long-term mental health disorders do not qualify for exclusion from these charges, and affordability and exemption status are issues that require attention when making enquiries regarding the availability of a service user's medication (Schafheutle, 2006). These are all considerations to make when setting the optimum conditions for pharmacological treatment.

7.   I am supported by my family, friends and doctor to take my medication

Family members (whether they are living together or not) and the social network can have an influential effect on an individual's treatment decisions and medication taking. As roles and relationships develop in response to mental health problems, attitudes and values can change with the result of coercion to either take or abstain from medication or the development of positive strategies that empower the service user's role in decision-making (Rogers et al., 1998). Where the person suffers from depression, relatives have voiced the need for information about the condition itself and treatment (Boyle & Chambers, 2000; Bollini et al., 2004). In a study which informed service users about tardive dyskinesia (TD), the authors concluded that although it was safer to inform people about the complication, telling them after treatment had been in place for some time risked alarm and anger in service users and relatives (Chaplin & Kent, 1998).

Agreement with service users should be reached regarding the limit of information that carers can be given regarding their illness and treatment. The *Mental Health Carers' Charter* (National Institute for Mental Health England, 2004) makes explicit six principles which enable the role of carers to be acknowledged and their needs to be met. Details in the charter include:

- It should be recognised that carers hold a special expertise in the condition of the person they are supporting, and their views should be sought and form part of the decision-making process. The distress that may be a result of this caring role needs to be addressed and the limits of their involvement should be respected.
- Details of the service user's mental health problem and treatment should be provided in a timely way and in the format which is most helpful.
- Carers should take an active role in planning and agreeing care plans. Incorporating their evaluation of how these treatment plans are working is good practice in the care process.

- The needs of the carers themselves require recognition and address; this includes their other commitments, and familial, cultural and personal factors.
- Carers require access to support, in terms of care planning and information about local groups, advocacy services and training opportunities as well as information about housing, employment and finances.
- Carers require the opportunity to influence and evaluate service development:

8.   I have a psychiatric disorder that antipsychotic medication improves

Insight is a complex, poorly understood and controversial area in the field of mental health, with lack of insight an often-quoted rationale for poor treatment adherence and engagement with services. It has been suggested that people with psychosis can develop two reactions to illness: a 'sealing-over' or denial, where a coping mechanism is put in place to reduce the feelings of stigma and overwhelming realisation of the person's circumstances, or, in contrast, a recovery style which seeks to understand and actively cope with illness, which has been referred to as an 'integrative' style (McGlashan et al., 1977). A study by Tait et al. (2003) suggests that people with a 'sealing over' recovery style were less likely to engage with services and that this way of dealing with illness occurred as symptoms improved and awareness of personal circumstances became clearer, unlike the acute phase of illness when a focus is maintained on becoming well and reducing distress. Recognising this and providing early support and information is an important aspect of acute care.

The author suggests that the interventions used in 'compliance therapy' (Kemp et al., 1996) may be effective by working with the person's psychological coping strategies to illness rather than addressing insight *per se*, although this study does have limitations and has not been successfully replicated.

Information giving

A significant part of medicines management is the provision of information, not only about the prescribed medications but also about the condition they are prescribed for and alternative treatments. Information giving is a crucial aspect of care as it provides the foundation for decision-making and therefore forms the basis of informed consent. In order for service users to develop hope and optimism for the future and mastery over their symptoms and relapse, information can guide them to use medication in recovery-orientated goals, making informed decisions about their treatment. Providing service users with an understanding of what they can expect from treatment facilitates the decision-making process, enabling them to weigh the pros and cons of suggested regimens.

The delivery of information must be undertaken in a planned and considered manner, adopting an interactive style in which the service users can feel comfortable to interrupt and ask questions, clarify issues and develop their knowledge. Flexibility should be built into informa-tion-giving sessions and the practitioner needs to be mindful of the duration of individual sessions and developing the level of detail and complexity of the information provided. A package can be constructed which gives general information, supplemented with leaflets and DVDs, and incorporates more information specific to the person's circumstances and regimen.

Facilitating the person's knowledge about medication should be seen as a practice which begins during the acute phase, when medica-tion is perhaps prescribed for the first time, and continues during follow-up meetings and care provided by community services. Infor-mation-giving should not be seen as a one-off event but continuous as the person develops greater understanding of his or her treatment and psychological experiences. It should also, where appropriate, involve the carers or relatives of service users, as their understanding of the issues can be critical in developing their opinions about the value of treatment and having informed discussions with their partner, relative or friend. In circumstances where confidentiality is an issue, informa-tion can be given from a more general perspective without reference to the service user's specific details.

Conclusion

Working with people and establishing their medication requirements is a collaborative process where the service users' views are vital in enabling the most effective regimen to be prescribed and to increase the probability a regimen will be prescribed which the person agrees to take. Work in this area is about providing information in a way which is best suited to individuals, ensuring they understand the ratio-nale for the prescription, and the actions and side effects of the drugs in order to make an informed decision about their medication require-ments. Where the service users agree, this process is also extended to their partner, relative or friends. Finding a medication regimen that the individuals find useful takes time; it involves assessment, monitoring and the implementation of interventions that help them achieve their goals and aspirations. The crucial aspect of achieving the optimum pharmaceutical treatment is the relationship built between the practitioner and service user: open, honest and genuinely collaborative.

References

Bollini, P., Tibaldi, G., Testa, C. & Munizza, C. (2004) Understanding treatment adherence in affective disorders; a qualitative study. *Journal of Psychiatric and Mental Health Nursing*, **11**, 668–674.

Boyle, E. & Chambers, M. (2000) Medication compliance in older individuals with depression; gaining the views of family carers. *Journal of Psychiatric and Mental Health Nursing*, **7**, 515–522.

Bryne, M.K., Deane, F. & Coombs, T. (2005) Nurses' beliefs and knowledge about medications are associated with their difficulties using patient treatment adherence strategies. *Journal of Mental Health*, **14**(5), 513–521.

Burton, S.C. (2005) Strategies for improving adherence to second generation antipsychotics in patients with schizophrenia by increasing ease of use. *Journal of Psychiatric Practice*, **11**, 369–378.

Chaplin, R. & Kent, A. (1998) Informing patients about tardive dyskinesia. *British Journal of Psychiatry*, **172**, 78–81.

Conley, R. & Buchanan, R. (1997) Evaluation of treatment-resistant schizophrenia. *Schizophrenia Bulletin*, **23**, 663–674.

Corrigan, P.W. (2002) Adherence to antipsychotic medications and health behaviour theories *Journal of Mental Health*, **11**, 243–254.

Day, J., Bentall, R., Roberts, C., et al. (2005) Attitude toward antipsychotic medication: The impact of clinical variables and relationships with health professionals. *Archives of General Psychiatry*, **62**, 717–724.

Demyttenaere, K. (1998) Non-compliance with antidepressants: Who's to blame? *International Clinical Psychopharmacology*, **13**, 19–25.

Dolder, C.R., Lacro, J.P., Warren, K.A., Golshan, S., Perkins, D.O. & Jeste, D.V. (2004) Brief evaluation of medication influences and beliefs: development and testing of a brief scale for medication adherence. *Journal of Clinical Psychopharmacology*, **24**, 404–409.

Fenton, W.S., Blyler, C.R. & Heinssen, R.K. (1997) Determinants of medication compliance in schizophrenia: empirical and clinical findings. *Schizophrenia Bulletin*, **23**(4), 637–651.

Haynes, R.B. (1976) A critical review of the determinants of patients compliance with therapeutic regimens. In: Sackett, D.L., Haynes, R.B. & Taylor, D.W. (eds) *Compliance with Therapeutic Regimens*. John Hopkins University Press, Baltimore.

Hornung, W.P., Klingberg, S., Feldmann, R., Schonauer, K. & Schulze Monking, H. (1998) Collaboration with drug treatment by schizophrenic patients with and without psychoeducational training: results of a 1-year follow-up. *Acta Psychiatrica Scandinavica*, **97**, 213–219.

Kemp, R., Heyward, P., Applewaite, G., Everitt, B. & David, A. (1996) Compliance therapy in psychotic patients; a randomised controlled trial. *British Medical Journal*, **312**, 345–349.

Lacro, J.P., Dunn, L.B., Dolder, C.R., Leckband, S.G. & Jeste, D.V. (2002) Prevalence of and risk factors for medication nonadherence in patients with schizophrenia: a comprehensive review of recent literature. *Journal of Clinical Psychiatry*, **63**, 892–909.

Ley, P. & Llewellyn, S. (1995) Improving patient's' understanding, recall, satisfaction and compliance. In: Bloome, A. & Llewellyn, S. (eds) *Health Psychology: Process and* Application. Croom, London.

Lieberman, J.A., Stroup, T.S., McEvoy, J.P., et al. (2005) Effectiveness of antipsychotic drugs in patients with chronic schizophrenia. *New England Journal of Medicine*, **353**(12), 1209–23.

Lindstrom, E. & Bingefors, K. (2000) Patient compliance with drug therapy in schizophrenia: economic and clinical issues. *Pharmacoeconomics*, **2**, 105–124.

Lingam, R. & Scott, J. (2002). Treatment non-adherence in affective disorders. *Acta Psychiatrica Scandinvica*, **105**(3), 164–172.

McGlashan, T.H., Wadeson, H.S., Carpenter, W.T., William, T. & Levy, S.T. (1977) Art and recovery style from psychosis. *Journal of Nervous and Mental Disease* **164**, 182–190.

Merinker, M. & Shaw, J. (2003) Not to be taken as directed; putting concordance for taking medicines into practice. *British Medical Journal*, **326**, 348–349.

Mueser, K.T., Corrigan, P.W. & Hilton, D.W. (2002) Illness management and recovery; a review of the research. *Psychiatric Services*, **53**, 1272–1284.

Müller, M.J. (2006) Attitudes toward different formulations of psychotropic drugs. The views of patients and healthcare providers. *American Journal of Drug Delivery*, **4**(1), 33–41.

National Institute for Mental Health England (2004) *The NIHME Mental Health Carers' Charter; Valuing Carers*. National Institute for Mental Health England, London.

National Institute for Mental Health England (2005) *Guiding Statement on Recovery*. National Institute for Mental Health England, London.

National Prescribing Centre (2007) *A Competency Framework for Shared Decision-making with Patients; Achieving Concordance for taking Medicines*. National Prescribing Centre, Keele.

Nursing and Midwifery Council (2004) *The NMC Code of Professional Conduct: Standards for Conduct, Performance and Ethics*. Nursing Midwifery Council, London.

Oehl, M., Hummer, M. & Fleischhacker, W.W. (2000) Compliance with antipsychotic treatment. *Acta Psychiatrica Scandinavica*, **S407**, 83–86.

Perkins, D.O. (1999) Adherence to antipsychotic medications. *Journal of Clinical Psychiatry*, **60**(S21), 25–30.

Perkins, D.O. (2002) Predictors of noncompliance in patients with schizophrenia. *Journal of Clinical Psychiatry*, **63**(12), 1121–8.

Rogers, A., Day, J.C., Williams, B., et al. (1998) The meaning and management of neuroleptic medication: a study of patients with a diagnosis of schizophrenia. *Social Science and Medicine*, **47**, 1313–1323.

Rosenstock, I.M. (1975) The Health Belief Model: explaining health behavior through expectancies. In: Glanz, K., Lewis, F.M. & Rimer, B.K. (eds) *Health Behavior and Health Education. Theory, Research and Practice*. Jossey-Bass, San Francisco, CA.

Schafheutle, E.I. (2006) Removing prescription charges for patients with mental health disorders: would it improve patient outcomes in the UK? *Disease Management and Health Outcomes*, **14**(3), 139–145.

Tait, L., Birchwood, M. & Trower, P. (2003) Predicting engagement with services for psychosis; insight symptoms and recovery style. *British Journal of Psychiatry*, **182**, 123–128.

Verdoux, H., Lengronne, J., Liraud, F. et al. (2000) Medication adherence in psychosis: predictors and impact on outcome: a 2-year follow-up of first-admitted patients. *Acta Psychiatrica Scandinavica*, **102**, 203–210.

Woodbridge, K. & Fulford, K.W.M. (2004) Whose values? A workbook for values-based practice in mental health care. Sainsbury Centre for Mental Health, London.

7

The negotiation of prescribing decisions: some good practice issues

Alan Quirk, Rob Chaplin, Paul Lelliott and Clive Seale

Introduction

There is considerable variation in the outcomes achieved for people with the same mental disorder who are offered the same treatment. These differences are in all domains of outcome, including alleviation of symptoms, functional improvement such as in ability to work and socialise, and in the need for future care, including hospitalisation. Some of this variation is caused by factors to do with the person, such as personality, severity and nature of symptoms, or degree of support; some is due to differences in the quality of the interaction between the service user and the practitioner(s). There is considerable evidence that a good therapeutic alliance is associated with better outcomes for people with serious mental illness (Howgego et al., 2003; McCabe & Priebe, 2004, 2008). At its extreme, poor service user–practitioner interaction manifests as disengagement and non-adherence. However, lesser degrees of impairment of the therapeutic alliance may also adversely affect outcomes by compromising the delivery of evidence-based treatments.

Although this most obviously applies to psychological therapies where the therapist–service user alliance is an overtly acknowledged therapeutic tool, the quality of the prescriber–service user relationship is also likely to affect the delivery of interventions that involve psychotropic drugs. This is reflected in the fact that user involvement in antipsychotic drug decisions is advocated in treatment guidelines (e.g. National Institute for Clinical Excellence, 2002; American Psychiatric

133

Association, 2004) and is thought to be integral to good psychiatric practice (Royal College of Psychiatrists, 2004; Bhugra & Holdsgrove, 2005).

This chapter reports on two studies of how such prescribing decisions are made. The first consists of interviews with 21 consultant psychiatrists about their experiences of consultations involving discussion of antipsychotic medication. The second is a series of 92 tape-recorded outpatient appointments with nine consultant psychiatrists. The recordings were transcribed and analysed using methods of conversation analysis in order to give a detailed insight into the interactions (Ten Have, 1999).

Although our studies only involved psychiatrists, our analysis is relevant to interactions involving non-medical prescribers, care-coordinators, keyworkers and named nurses in secondary care, and, when prescribing takes place in primary care, discussions between general practitioners (GPs) and other mental health practitioners. This is because people undertaking these roles may also be present at the consultation and may indeed have set up the meeting with a desired outcome. Doctors are also care-coordinators and share generic mental health skills (for example relationship building, empathy, listening skills, provision of information). These will be important to all professionals who work alongside people with psychosis. Finally, non-medical mental health workers are increasingly taking a lead in decisions about users' medication as psychiatrists adopt new working practices and review fewer service users routinely.

This chapter begins by examining shared decision-making, as practised in psychiatric outpatient consultations. Our analysis reveals that shared decision-making is highly variable, with some shared decisions being a great deal more 'shared' than others. We then consider how service users' concerns about feeling drowsy and lethargic ('like a zombie') on antipsychotic medication are sometimes engaged with by psychiatrists, but more often not. The remainder of the chapter considers a consultation that began with a service user reporting that he had been experiencing seizures. This triggered a prescribing decision (to swap antipsychotics), which has features that illuminate issues of general relevance to prescribing practice. By combining findings from in-depth interviews with psychiatrists with observation of real-life practice (taped outpatient consultations), we aim to discuss good practice issues with an understanding of the everyday challenges and dilemmas faced by practitioners.

Shared decision-making in practice

Shared decision-making is generally thought to be characterised by participants sharing information, taking steps to build a consensus and reaching an explicit agreement on the treatment to be implemented (Charles et al., 1997). While such an approach is increasingly being advocated, there has been very little research about its use in mental health care. Most research has been about primary care interactions. Our interview study (Seale et al., 2006) explored this issue and found that most psychiatrists aspired to shared decision-making. The majority, when working in routine outpatient consultations (16/21), felt there had been a trend toward 'patient-centred' practice, with 14/21 preferring a cooperative relationship with shared decision-making, negotiated agreements and a sense of partnership. However, these psychiatrists also felt that implementing shared decision-making was difficult with service users who lacked insight. It was also acknowledged that the power psychiatrists have (e.g. to invoke mental health legislation) can be perceived by service users as militating against a truly shared approach, and that this makes psychiatry different from other areas of medicine. Although psychiatrists acknowledged the need for firmer or more directive styles, for example when a person was relapsing, lacking insight or at risk, they were concerned about the damaging effects of this type of approach on the future therapeutic alliance and reverted to shared decision-making as soon as possible.

Our analysis of outpatient transcripts identified the extent to which service users and psychiatrists achieved their desired outcomes with regard to antipsychotic prescribing (Quirk, 2007a,b). Change was actively sought by the user and/or psychiatrist in 43 of the 92 consultations. Similar proportions of consultants (14/21) and users (16/22) achieved their 'preferred' prescribing decision outcomes (such as dose increases/reductions, swapping from one antipsychotic to another or stopping the antipsychotic altogether). This evidence for balance in the negotiations ties in with these psychiatrists' self-image of 'patient-centeredness'.

That noted, our analysis looked beyond who achieved their desired prescribing outcome to examine *how* the prescribing decisions were made. In doing so it was possible to observe that some shared decisions are considerably more 'shared' than others. At one extreme we observed service users being allowed to decide about their medication, with the psychiatrist exerting no pressure on the decision-making either way. These types of decisions are likely to arise in situations where alternative treatments (or no treatment) are perceived by the psychiatrist to have similar outcomes in terms of benefits or risks, and where a person is judged to have capacity to make such choices. And at the other extreme we saw psychiatrists exerting pressure such that the service user had very little option other than to go along with what the psychiatrist clearly wanted. Although the outcome was typically agreed and 'consensus' was achieved, it is clear to everyone involved that it had been the psychiatrist's decision. These decisions perhaps run a risk of not being acted on by service users, resulting in non-adherence, although longitudinal studies would be needed to confirm this.

When there is a disagreement about treatment, alternative strategies to exerting pressure should be considered. These were explored in the analysis by Chaplin et al. (2007) of the psychiatrists' interview study. These might include giving the service user information and allowing more time for him or her to decide by rescheduling an appointment, striking a bargain about another issue (e.g. stopping cannabis use), tolerating disagreement and accepting that applying pressure might lead to a loss of face for either party.

Engaging with service users' concerns

Sedation and mental clouding caused by antipsychotic medication may contribute to social withdrawal. However, the severity of this side effect of medication may be underestimated by psychiatrists. In a survey of more than 2000 service users (National Schizophrenia Fellowship, 2001), sedation and lethargy were the most common complaint of respondents and reported to be the worst adverse effect associated with taking medication for mental illness. The analysis of quantitative data from our observational study of outpatient consultations also found that sedation and mental clouding were the side effects that users were most concerned about (Seale et al., 2007). Although service users raised this issue in 37 of the 92 consultations, sometimes on more than one occasion, psychiatrists only mentioned it independently in eight consultations. Psychiatrists were much more concerned about potential blood changes brought about by antipsychotic medication (raised 47 times by psychiatrists but only 16 times by service users). These included the need to monitor levels of blood sugar, cholesterol or lipids, often with regard to concerns about developing diabetes. It appears that psychiatrists and service users had different priorities with regard to the types of side effects attended to in these meetings.

Psychiatrists did not seem to be good at responding to reports of sedation and mental clouding when presented by the user as troublesome (as opposed to, say, a welcome part of normal experience). Indeed, there were only three instances where the psychiatrist directly engaged with such concerns. One attempt evidently caused the service user some discomfort, and this was where the psychiatrist challenged his medication-taking behaviour ('so why do you take [your antipsychotic] during the day if it makes you drowsy'). The other two, more successful, attempts were where the psychiatrist engaged in sympathetic and supportive listening, and where the psychiatrist carefully listened to the person's concerns and offered helpful advice, namely to take the medication at night, 'because some people do find these helpful, making sure you get to sleep and it can still do all its antipsychotic work as well'. In all other cases, feeling drowsy was either marked as positive (e.g. by the psychiatrist responding that taking the tablet 'must help' with sleep), or denied or avoided (e.g. by the psychiatrist questioning the service user's interpretation of the experience, or changing the subject).

This behaviour by psychiatrists is similar to that described by another observational study of psychiatric outpatient consultations (McCabe et al., 2002). Here, psychiatrists showed a reluctance to respond to people talking about the content of their psychotic symptoms. Service users actively attempted to do this, for example by asking direct questions and repeating questions and utterances. In response the psychiatrists hesitated, responded with a question rather than an answer, and smiled or laughed (when informal carers were present), indicating their reluctance to engage with service users' concerns. For example, when one person asked 'Why don't people believe me when I say I'm God', the psychiatrist responded with a question: 'What should I say now?' and laughter. The authors argue that this is a typical response, although they also warn against generalising from the few selected cases examined in their paper (McCabe et al., 2002).

Combined, the findings from these two observational studies of psychiatric outpatient consultations offer good evidence for how psychiatrists may *block communication* about issues they regard as being irrelevant to matters in hand. It follows that psychiatrists, and possibly other mental health professionals, need to focus on improving their listening skills and their ability to attend and respond to service users' concerns. The use of structured rating instruments to measure self-reported side effects, for example the Liverpool University Neuroleptic Side Effect Rating Scale (Day et al., 1995) scale, is likely to improve the detection of side effects and provide healthcare professionals and service users with opportunities to focus on each one.

Case example: a negotiated prescribing decision

In a small number of the consultations we observed, a prescribing decision was triggered by the service user reporting his or her experience of side effects. A summary of the content of one such consultation is presented (Box 7.1). In this example the service user (SU) and consultant psychiatrist (C) quickly arrived at a shared understanding of the seriousness of the situation (the service user reported he had been experiencing fits) and of the need to do something about it. A small part of the consultation – the exchange highlighted in bold – will be examined in more detail later in the chapter.

Box 7.1 Summary of consultation 50

Duration – 24 minutes

Outcome – Swapping of antipsychotics (from olanzapine to sulpiride)

In response to an opening question by the consultant (C), the service user (SU) reports having been 'not so well' lately because he has had an 'epilepsy thing' (experiencing seizures). Service user reports not knowing if it had had anything to do with the medication he has been taking (olanzapine).

After exploring exactly what had happened, C informs SU that all medication for psychosis lowers the threshold for seizures, and suggests that one option would be to stop the medication altogether. C then successfully persuades SU into agreeing to this.

After further discussion, C has second thoughts and checks for an alternative antipsychotic in the *British National Formulary* (*BNF*). After a lengthy pause while he refers to the book, C reports back that he recommends sulpiride as a less risky drug, regarding seizures, and offers three choices:

(a) to stop the medication,
(b) to cut down the dose of olanzapine, or
(c) to start on different medication at low dose.

C asks what SU would like to do; he chooses to try the new medication.

C informs SU about side effects of the new medication, then reaffirms that the best thing is to stop the olanzapine straight away. C writes a prescription and apologises to SU for what has happened. SU asks if he can finish his medication. C says no, 'I wouldn't take any more of that', and says that SU should 'go for your choice and take a different medication'.

C explains that ordinarily he'd get SU to take both antipsychotics at the same for a while to help the transition from one to the other, but 'we can't do that because that would make you more likely to have a fit'.

After advising SU when and how to take the new medication, and discussing with SU how he is doing at university, C repeats that SU should stop his present antipsychotic immediately, then closes the consultation.

Few advocates of shared decision-making would argue that it is appropriate in every clinical situation. In crisis situations there is often little time for the healthcare professional to build a consensus with the service user about what should be done, and this is compounded in situations where a person's capacity to make informed decisions about the treatment is in question (discussed further in Seale et al., 2006). The classic paper by Szasz and Hollender (1955) on different models of the 'doctor–patient' relationship is perhaps helpful for interpreting the consultation summarised above. This concludes that the model of 'mutual participation' is only one of a number of possible doctor–patient relationships. Others include 'activity–passivity', where the doctor does something to the completely helpless service user, and 'guidance–cooperation', where the person with an acute condition seeks help and is ready to cooperate. It is important that the mental healthcare practitioner recognises that there are these different types of professional–client relationship or interactional styles and even consciously applies or adapts a selected style that fits the particular encounter with a service user.

Returning to Consultation 50 (Box 7.1), it can be seen that the service user sought help and cooperated with the guidance offered, so it is probably best categorised as conforming to a 'guidance–cooperation' approach. Arguably, this is a good example of the type of situation where it is entirely appropriate to adopt a more directive style, as it required the doctor to use his expertise to assist the person in choosing a comparatively safer prescribing option.

Our analysis of this consultation does not end here. Precisely *how* was the service user guided such that he chose the drug evidently preferred by the consultant? In the next section we will look at just one of the techniques used.[1]

Delivering information about adverse effects: How much, and when?

Research studies indicate that there are different views and perceptions about the quality of communication about adverse effects of medication in psychiatric practice (Laugharne et al., 2004). Surveys of service users suggest that insufficient information is given (Mind, 1998; National Schizophrenia Fellowship, 2000; Olofinjana & Taylor, 2005). However, these studies are based on self reports by psychiatrists or service users, so they are subject to recall bias. This means it is possible that psychiatrists may be optimistic in their estimates of how much information they provide, while service users may forget what they have been told. Observational studies can answer this question by examining not only how much information about side effects is actually delivered in a given meeting or consultation, but also *when* it is delivered. To illustrate the importance of this issue, which has been neglected in the research literature to date, we will examine one instance, which occurred in the case example presented above. The

---

[1] A detailed conversation analysis of the transcript of this consultation may be found in Quirk (2007a). It will be also presented in a forthcoming publication.

Detailed extract from Consultation 50		
Duration of extract = 23 seconds		
Outcome = Swapping of anti-psychotics (from Olanzapine to Sulpiride)		
1	Consultant:	Wha- what d' you think you'd like [to do (about)
2	Service user:	[Well I think I-Iwould like to
3		try the new medica [tion
4	Consultant:	[Yeah
5	Service user:	(French) new medication ( )
6	Consultant:	Yeah .hhh the (0.2) I'm just trying to think the- possibly the
7		most (0.6) likely side effect are (0.6) yer sexual performance
8		might be affected by it (0.5) in terms of (0.2) delayed
9		ejaculation. (But) that's the most likely thing that can
10		happen (0.4) (that) doesn't happen with everybody
11		or [a lot of people
12	Service user:	[.hhh (fine) actually I am single so=

Figure 7.1   Detailed extract from Consultation 50.

transcript shown above (Figure 7.1) is a more detailed version of the exchange highlighted in the consultation summary (see Box 7.1): '*C asks what SU would like to do; he chooses to try the new medication*'.

The transcript uses conventions that allow the representation of some key features of speech delivery. These include intakes of breath ('.hhh'), pauses ('0.2' in brackets denotes a silence of 0.2 seconds), speaker emphasis (shown with underlining) and overlaps (shown with square brackets). Words in brackets are possible interpretations of speech that was not absolutely clear on tape, and empty brackets are words that could not be made out.

Two key observations may be made for present purposes. The first is about when the information about side effects is delivered by the consultant. Notice how this is done, on lines 6–11, only after the service user has already chosen to swap antipsychotics, on lines 2–3 (this was the first time that side effects of sulpiride were discussed in this consultation). This does not conform to models of informed decision-making which assume such information is delivered before the service user decides. The second observation is that the consultant delivers information on one potential side effect only – delayed ejaculation (lines 8–9) – rather than, say, the three or four most likely side effects. Without presenting the full analysis (see Quirk, 2007a,b), it can be observed that these actions function to reinforce the decision, and certainly do not encourage the service user to change his mind about trying the new medication.

Thus, minimal information is delivered only after the service user has chosen a different antipsychotic, and at a point in the decision-making when it would be difficult to revise his choice. Does this amount to bad practice? Viewed out of context, one would have to conclude that it is. However, further scrutiny of this small piece of data reveals a simple method sometimes used by psychiatrists to 'solve' one of their central dilemmas.

Conversational solution to a central dilemma for psychiatrists

Our interview study (Seale et al., 2006) identified a central dilemma for psychiatrists, namely that while most are convinced about the value of antipsychotic medications, they worry about the consequences of fully explaining adverse effects for fear of compromising adherence to prescribing.[2] Also, psychiatrists mentioned the difficulty in providing comprehensive or precise information about side effects. This is because these drugs have very many potential side effects, some of which are extremely rare. It would be impractical, and possibly alarmist, to discuss all of these. Also, any combination of side effects, or none, may be experienced by an individual.

In the transcript (Figure 7.1) we can observe the consultant applying one particular conversational solution to this dilemma which, in this specific context, reinforces the decision to swap antipsychotics. The key to this is in how the consultant refers only to the *'most likely'* side effect of the new medication and glosses over the rest (line 7). By specifying in advance the precise number of side effects about which information will be imparted (in this case 'most likely' = 1, although the consultant might have chosen to discuss, say, the 'top three'), this allows a doctor to imply there are other adverse effects *without having to say what they are.* In turn, this puts the onus onto the service users to request further information should they feel they need it (which in this case he chooses not to do). Thus, the consultant is able to impart only a very limited amount of information about side effects, but in a manner that is not overtly misleading (compared with not mentioning side effects at all, or denying that the drug has any adverse effects). Further, in *ranking* side effects by their likelihood or importance, the psychiatrist invokes his or her expertise. This is a more sophisticated approach than, say, referring to the *BNF* and dutifully reading out every single side effect to the service user. It is likely that service users will have more faith in the implicit knowledge of the consultant – even though they have been given incomplete information. In other words, it is a

[2]Communication about adherence to prescribing is examined in Quirk (2007b) and will be the subject of a forthcoming paper.

method in and through which mental healthcare professionals can deliver minimal information, and quickly, such that it conveys they are 'prioritising' what the service user really needs to know. Clearly, there is a risk of this being interpreted as the professional withholding information about the many other possible side effects, but that was evidently not so in this example.

Conclusion

The therapeutic alliance and the style of interaction between psychiatrist and service user influence outcomes independent of treatment modality. Our interviews and observational study were restricted to psychiatrist and service user interactions (although other mental healthcare professionals were sometimes involved in the consultations). Other limitations were the small sample of psychiatrists involved and the possible lack of representativeness of practices in other centres or countries. Moreover, there was only one measure of 'proximal' outcome, i.e. the outcome at the end of the session. Further research should involve a wider variety of mental health professionals and use longitudinal measures of outcome.

Overall these studies confirm the importance of empathy, of anticipating and eliciting a service user's views and of listening skills, especially those regarding side effects and symptoms. They suggest that shared decision-making, as practised in psychiatric outpatient consultations, covers a range of interactional styles, with some decisions being more 'shared' than others. The findings show that psychiatrists do adopt different interactional styles in different circumstances that range from offering service users a free choice to being highly directive. Psychiatrists sometimes underestimate or avoid service users' concerns, noticeably those related to feeling drowsy and lethargic on antipsychotic medication. Given the value that users place on these types of adverse effect, this might be an important contributor to future non-adherence.

The ability to 'get on with' people who may not have insight, have poor concentration, or may be reluctant to be engaged with care is an essential skill for those working in mental health. Despite this, many practitioners have very few opportunities to receive objective feedback about their communication skills. This is something that should be addressed, for example by providing opportunities for practitioners to observe, and be observed by, colleagues interacting with service users and to provide and receive feedback. Multidisciplinary working should facilitate this practice and is favoured over working in isolation. By revealing what other practitioners do, observational studies such as ours can help people working in mental health to reflect on their own practice.

Acknowledgements

The authors would like to thank the service users and psychiatrists involved in the study. We would also like to thank the funder of the study, Eli Lilly, who did not influence the conduct of the research.

References

American Psychiatric Association (2004) *Practice Guideline for the Treatment of Patients with Schizophrenia.* American Psychiatric Association, Washington, DC.

Bhugra, D. & Holsgrove, G. (2005) Patient-centred psychiatry, training and assessment: the way forward. *Psychiatric Bulletin*, **29**, 49–52.

Chaplin, R., Lelliott, P., Quirk, A. & Seale, C. (2007) Negotiating styles adopted by consultant psychiatrists when prescribing antipsychotics. *Advances in Psychiatric Treatment*, **13**, 43–50.

Charles, C.A., Gafni, A. & Whelan, T. (1997) Shared decision-making in the medical encounter: what does it mean? (Or it takes at least two to tango). *Social Science and Medicine*, **44**(5), 681–692.

Day, J., Wood, G., Dewey, M. & Bentall, R.P. (1995) A self-rating scale for measuring neuroleptic side-effects: Validation in a group of schizophrenic patients. *British Journal of Psychiatry*, **166**, 650–653.

Howgego, I.M., Yellowlees, P., Owen, C., Meldrum, L. & Dark, F. (2003) The therapeutic alliance: the key to effective patient outcome? A descriptive review of the evidence in community mental health case management. *Australian and New Zealand Journal of Psychiatry*, **37**(2), 169–183.

Laugharne, J., Davies, A., Arcelus, J. & Bouman, W.P. (2004) Informing patients about tardive dyskinesia: a survey of clinicians' attitudes in three countries. *International Journal of Law and Psychiatry*, **27**(1), 101–108.

McCabe, R. & Priebe, S. (2004) The therapeutic relationship in the treatment of severe mental illness: a review of methods and findings. *International Journal of Social Psychiatry*, **50**(2), 115–128.

McCabe, R. & Priebe, S. (2008) Communication and psychosis: It's good to talk, but how? (Editorial). *British Journal of Psychiatry*, **192**, 404–405.

McCabe, R., Heath, C., Burns, T. & Priebe, S. (2002) Engagement of patients with psychosis in the consultation. *British Medical Journal*, **325**, 1148–1151.

Mind. (1998) *Psychiatric Drugs: Users' Experience and Current Policy and Practice.* Mind, London.

National Institute for Clinical Excellence (2002) *Schizophrenia: Core Interventions in the Treatment and Management of Schizophrenia in Primary and Secondary Care*. National Institute for Clinical Excellence, London.

National Schizophrenia Fellowship (2000) *A Question of Choice*. National Schizophrenia Fellowship, London.

National Schizophrenia Fellowship (2001) *Doesn't It Make You Sick?* National Schizophrenia Fellowship, London..

Olofinjana, B. & Taylor, D. (2005) Antipsychotic drugs – information and choice: a patient survey. *Psychiatric Bulletin*, **29**, 369–371.

Quirk, A. (2007a) How pressure is applied in 'negotiated' decisions about medication. In: *Obstacles to shared decision-making in psychiatric practice: findings from three observational studies*. PhD thesis, Brunel University, Uxbridge.

Quirk, A. (2007b) Communication about adherence to long-term anti-psychotic prescribing. In: *Obstacles to shared decision-making in psychiatric practice: findings from three observational studies*. PhD thesis, Brunel University, Uxbridge.

Royal College of Psychiatrists (2004) *Good Psychiatric Practice*. 2nd edn. CR125. Royal College of Psychiatrists, London.

Seale, C., Chaplin, R., Lelliott, P. & Quirk, A. (2006) Sharing decisions in consultations involving antipsychotic medication: a qualitative study of psychiatrists' experiences. *Social Science & Medicine*, **62**, 2861–2873.

Seale, C., Chaplin, R., Lelliott, P. & Quirk, A. (2007) Antipsychotic medication, sedation and mental clouding: An observational study of psychiatric consultations. *Social Science and Medicine*, **65**, 698–711.

Szasz, T.S. & Hollender, T.S. (1955) A contribution to the philosophy of medicine: the basic models of the doctor–patient relationship. *Archives of Internal Medicine*, **97**(5): 585—592.

Ten Have, P. (1999) *Doing Conversation Analysis: A Practical Guide*. Sage, London.

The role of the pharmacy in medicines management

David Branford and Peter Pratt

Introduction

In this chapter, we will describe how pharmacy services are organised, structured and delivered for mental health. We will examine the background reports and guidance that are currently shaping the development of future pharmacy services, identifying priorities and changing practice. The services provided by pharmacy departments across the full spectrum of healthcare provision and how mental health medicines management is integrated within this context will be described. The roles and responsibilities of pharmacy staff will be discussed along with new innovations in practice.

Definition of medicines management in the context of pharmacy

In 2001, the Audit Commission adopted the term 'medicines management' in its report *A Spoonful of Sugar – Medicines Management in NHS Hospitals* to encompass:

> *'The entire way that medicines are selected, procured, delivered, prescribed, administered and reviewed to optimise the contribution that medicines make to produce informed and desired outcomes of patient care.'*

Audit Commission (2001)

Although focusing initially on acute hospitals, this emphasised the fact that good medicines use cannot occur in isolation. Multiple processes are involved, all linked under the over-arching term of 'medicines management'.

For mental health trusts (MHTs), the publication of the *Spoonful of Sugar* document began a process of examination, looking at the infrastructures needed to support good medicines management. This review took place against an increased concern that many MHTs were weak in this area. The initiatives started by the Audit Commission were followed up by the Healthcare Commission (2007a), who published a report on medicines management in mental health called *Talking about medicines. The management of medicines in trusts providing mental health services.*

Talking about medicines identified that leadership is central to the successful development of 10 focus areas for medicines management. These are:

- involving people in decisions regarding the management of their medicines;
- ensuring appropriate and effective use of medicines in people's care;
- efficiently and effectively providing and administering medicines;
- promoting multidisciplinary team working to provide seamless care;
- coordinating care with other providers;
- governing the use of medicines;
- choosing and prescribing medicines;
- ensuring staff are competent to work with medicines;
- accurately recording and reporting on the use of medicines;
- supplying and managing medicines in the trust.

Leading and developing this agenda is a core activity for pharmacy staff employed by MHTs.

Clearly, medicines management is not just about pharmacists – or pharmacy staff in general. Medicines management in mental health cannot be achieved by any professional group working in isolation. To succeed in providing a high quality service it is important to recognise that mental health pharmacists, and other pharmacy staff, are an integral part of service delivery, providing leadership, skills and expertise in medicines management. The wider agenda includes practitioners becoming skilled in the use of medicines and achieving good outcomes for their service users through the techniques of medicines management.

Organisation of pharmacy services for mental health, primary care trusts and secondary care

Community pharmacies

Community pharmacists are primarily employed as independent contractors. In general terms they are either owner-contractors (they own and manage the community pharmacy) or employees of a company-contractor (e.g. Boots) and are contracted to the NHS to dispense medicines. The majority of their pharmacy-related employment comes from dispensing medicines detailed in prescriptions written by prescribers, who are predominantly general practitioners (GPs). In recent years, community pharmacists have been encouraged to develop additional enhanced services, such as dispensing in 'blister' or dosette packs, and changes to the contract for community pharmacists have provided methods of payment for these additional roles. Most of the medicines for mental health and learning disabilities services users are dispensed in community pharmacies. Community pharmacists are a primary source of general medicines information and provide assistance to both service users and community nurses (Healthcare Commission, 2007b).

Primary care trust pharmacists

Primary care trust (PCT) pharmacists fall into a number of categories:

- pharmacy advisors, who have wide ranging responsibilities to oversee the use of medicines across the whole PCT, including mental health drugs. This role has recently been divided into commissioner and provider roles;
- practice pharmacists, who work with one or a number of GPs to assist them with the use of medicines in their practice(s);
- pharmacists, who provide services to PCT facilities and specialties such as small general hospitals or specialist clinics.

Many PCT GP practice pharmacists are being encouraged to become non-medical prescribers or pharmacists with a special interest (Department of Health, 2006) and may undertake joint clinics with practice-based, nurse non-medical prescribers.

Secondary care pharmacists

The secondary care mental health pharmacy workforce comprises four main groups: pharmacists, pharmacy technicians, pharmacy assistants (also called assistant technical officers, ATOs) and other ancillary and clerical staff.

Pharmacists

Pharmacists are a highly qualified group of staff undertaking a 4-year university-based masters degree followed by a 1-year pre-registration period to achieve registration with the Royal Pharmaceutical Society of Great Britain. Most hospital pharmacists undertake a further 2–3 years of clinical training to qualify to practise as a clinical pharmacist. Further qualifications in mental health pharmacy are also available at postgraduate certificate and diploma levels.

In 2000 the UK Psychiatric Pharmacy Group established the College of Mental Health Pharmacists (CMHP). To achieve membership of the CMHP, pharmacists need to demonstrate a high level of skills in the delivery of specialist mental health pharmacy services.

Pharmacy technicians (also called medicines management technicians)

Pharmacy technicians undertake 2–3 years of work-based training. In the past this has resulted in qualifications from Apothecary Hall, City and Guilds Institute, Business and Technological Education Council and currently National Vocational Qualification (NVQ) level 3. In recent years, foundation degree and diploma qualifications have developed for pharmacy technicians working within acute trusts and PCTs to facilitate the development of new ward and patient focus based roles. Pharmacy technicians undertake most of the dispensing and manufacturing duties in the pharmacy. In acute trusts, they have increasingly taken over the role of ordering stock and repeat medicines for wards.

Pharmacy assistants or assistant technical officers

Pharmacy assistants or assistant technical officers (ATOs) receive in-house training and undertake an NVQ qualification. Pharmacy assistants can undertake many of the routine medicine-related tasks in the pharmacy and increasingly on wards. They have been identified as a group who can develop new ways of working (NWW), allowing the release of pharmacy technicians to undertake more complex tasks and the release of ward nursing time from the routine ordering of medicines.

Clerical and other support staff

Pharmacists and pharmacy technicians are unlikely to be available to work as part of the clinical teams if the support infrastructures are not in place. Three examples of where new work has added to the clerical burden of the pharmacy are the administrative support for the Drugs and Therapeutics Committee (DTC), medicines audits and the supply and supervision of prescribing pads.

Mental health trust pharmacy services

The nature and size of the pharmacy service available to any MHT and the service it provides is dependent on a variety of factors, including:

1. the outcome for the pharmacy service following the closure of the mental institutions or asylums;
2. the extent to which specialist mental health pharmacy services were retained within the acute hospital environment;
3. the development of clinical pharmacy in mental health in the locality;
4. the leadership of a chief pharmacist for the MHT and the ability of that person to develop specialist mental health pharmacy services;
5. the recognition that community-based services will involve at least the same if not more specialist pharmacy services;
6. the level of support for specialist pharmacy services by the MHT board and commissioners.

In 2006, a survey was undertaken across England to ascertain the size and capacity of the MHT pharmacy workforce (Taylor & Sutton, 2006; Branford et al., 2006a,b). The key findings relating to MHT pharmacy services were as follows:

- Mental health trusts vary hugely in size and activity. They are different from other trusts in the extent to which medicines-related activities are devolved to others, such as community pharmacists, GPs and acute trusts, and this impacts on the priorities for MHT pharmacy services. This inevitably has an effect on the complexity of the MHT pharmacy services, which may be further complicated by operating over many sites.
- Most MHTs are dependent on other providers for their pharmacy services through the use of service level agreements (SLA). Only 17% provided their own pharmacy services, in contrast to 25% requiring three or more such agreements. The pattern of service delivery where 'the MHT has no pharmacy of its own and receives all aspects of the pharmacy service from another Trust' was the most common pattern for supply of pharmaceuticals (58%). However, the impact of SLAs is far greater than this with only 17% of the participating MHTs managing all their own supply services and 27% managing all their own clinical pharmacy services without requiring an SLA.

The ability of MHT pharmacy services to manage the process in which medicines are used by a trust depends on the availability of a pharmacy workforce. The survey identified that:

- Pharmacists represent a small workforce in mental health with only 371 whole time equivalents (WTE) employed by 59 MHTs in England.
- No 'formula' is used to match the size of the trust's catchment population with the number of pharmacists employed, with some very large MHTs employing only one or two per million population served and others employing 15–20 for a similar size of MHT. Five MHTs between them employed 100 of the pharmacists. Although there was a trend towards those MHTs very dependent on SLA employing fewer pharmacists in mental health, this was not always the case.
- The Sainsbury Centre for Mental Health (Boardman & Parsonage, 2007) has published a report suggesting the resources required for a 'good mental health service' for adults. Although it is difficult to extrapolate from such proposals, on the basis of the report the numbers of mental health pharmacists required may be of the order of three to four times the currently available workforce.
- Pharmacists have a key role to play in the management of medicines by MHTs and a great potential to undertake prescribing roles following the introduction of legislation for both supplementary and independent pharmacist prescribing. It is very difficult so see how these roles can develop with such low numbers of mental health pharmacists.
- Pharmacy technicians represent an even smaller workforce in mental health with only 270 WTE employed by 59 MHTs in England. The findings for pharmacy technicians mirror those for pharmacists.

Clinical pharmacy and the role of the specialist mental health clinical pharmacist

Before the 1960s, most psychiatric hospitals contained a pharmacy and employed one or more pharmacists; traditionally that pharmacist's role was to supply and manufacture medicines. The pharmacist was rarely involved in direct patient care. From the 1960s, concern about medicine errors and the increasing complexity of medicines led to a gradual change in the role and training of pharmacists within secondary care as a whole. Medicines have become more potent and more complex to prescribe. It has become more difficult for prescribers to keep abreast of all the changes and prescribing has become more of a team activity, requiring input from pharmacists.

It is now increasingly accepted within mental health and clinical practice that prescribing performance is enhanced and risks reduced by the inclusion of a specialist mental health clinical pharmacist within clinical teams. This has changed the pharmacist's role from a product-focused role to a service user focused role and has had enormous implications for the number of pharmacists required to provide such a service. However, despite this change occurring in most acute trusts, surveys of the pharmacy workforce have identified that in many MHTs modernisation of the pharmacists' role, where they are being entirely clinically focused within a ward/team-based role, has yet to occur.

In addition to these ward/team-based roles, specialist mental health clinical pharmacists monitor the use of medicines throughout an organisation with the aim of ensuring that service users receive clinically effective, cost-effective and, most importantly, safe medicines. The overall aim is to achieve best outcomes from pharmacological treatments with minimal side effects and adverse problems.

Much of mental health policy in recent times has been to move the focus of mental health care and treatment from hospitals into the community. The National Service Framework (NSF) for mental health recognised the skill deficit in many multidisciplinary teams around complex medication (Department of Health, 1999). It also set guidelines and targets for the development of crisis, home treatment and assertive outreach services to enhance an array of other community mental health teams. Unfortunately, little progress has been made to address the issue of complex medicines management in teams, and throughout the UK there has been little progress in employing specialist mental health pharmacists as team members.

Access to medicines information services varies from trust to trust. In some trusts there are no specific information services provided, whereas in others wards clinical staff are able to telephone the pharmacy department for detailed information about mental health medicines or have access to written material about medicines supplied and maintained by the pharmacy. Other trusts have developed forums about medicines for service users and carers, medicines websites and medicines helplines.

Medicines management schemes and interventions

In the Audit Commission's *Spoonful of Sugar* report, a number of schemes and programmes were identified that could improve the use of medicines by acute hospitals. These were prioritised to include recommendations regarding;

- greater involvement by MHT boards in overseeing medicines management;
- providing leadership for medicines management by a chief pharmacist;
- greater accountability and role for the drug & therapeutics committee (DTC) (or equivalent).

The Audit Commission also recommended a number of schemes relating to:

- the clinical role and responsibility of the pharmacists;
- admission and discharge schemes (both clinical and administrative areas have been identified as having high risk of medicines errors);
- self-medication schemes for service users in hospital;
- the use of patient's own drugs while in hospital;
- automation of supplies.

In many acute trusts a new system for managing service users' medicines on wards has been advocated. Called 'one-stop dispensing' it involves the following components:

- On admission to hospital (usually a planned admission) the service user or carer is asked to bring his or her own medicines.
- The suitability for continued use of the service user's medicines (referred to as 'patients' own drugs' or PODs) is assessed by pharmacy technicians or in some cases by specially trained nurses.
- Medicines reconciliation, which includes a drug history, is taken by the ward-based pharmacist or a specially trained technician to check the accuracy of the medicines against their prescription and review the need for the medicines. This may also involve liaison with the service user's GP and community pharmacist.
- Nurses either administer medicines from the service user's own supplies or use personalised stock medicines. Alternatively, service users self-administer their own medicines.
- Medicines are stored in individual bedside lockers to facilitate self-administration or individual lockers are located in one trolley overseen by a nurse.
- The individual supplies are used to assess the knowledge and skills of the service users to manage their own medicines.
- Preparation for discharge is achieved by pharmacy staff ensuring that the service user's locker contains sufficient medicines and that the service user is well informed about them.
- Rapid discharge is achieved by service users taking their own medicines with them on leaving hospital.

Most acute trusts have adopted new ways of working (NWW) initiatives to enable specially trained technicians (also called medicines management technicians) to undertake one-stop dispensing.

These recommendations, however, related to acute hospitals. In 2001 the Changing Workforce Programme for Mental Health invited the Newcastle, North Tyneside and Northumberland Mental Health Trust to develop and evaluate a programme of NWW in mental health pharmacy. The aim of the programme was to investigate the potential for the pharmacy to have a positive impact on the delivery of medicine-related services to mental health service users. This was to be achieved by developing the roles of pharmacy staff to create improved services to service users and to release time for other mental healthcare professionals to improve services and undertake work related to the management of medicines by service users.

The Spread Programme

Between 2002 and 2005 all MHTs in England were invited to participate in a programme of small innovations (the Spread Programme; Pratt & Branford, 2007) that demonstrated the potential of mental health pharmacy services to disseminate new medicines management practices to MHTs. Approximately half of the MHTs in England participated. A total of 38 different mental health sites submitted completed accounts of 40 projects. The details of the schemes and the report are available on the NWW website (www.newwaysofworking.org.uk).

The three fundamental findings in the report were:

- Schemes that allow better access to pharmacy staff for wards or community teams result in improved medicines management.
- Any project that places pharmacy staff as members of the clinical ward or community team is likely to improve relationships, improve medicines management and lead to better outcomes for service users.
- Many MHTs depend on acute trusts for their pharmacy services. Such services are organised to provide for the acute trust and are not always appropriate for the MHT.

Further supplementary findings were:

- Pharmacists and pharmacy services should not work in isolation.
- The reuse of PODs in mental health as a NWW is not generally financially self-supporting. However, aspects within the one-stop dispensing process, such as the review by pharmacy staff of service users' medicines on admission and the further integration of pharmacy staff with clinical teams, did have benefits for service users through improved systems of medicines management.

- The potential benefit of employing specialist pharmacists to work in review clinics was demonstrated.
- Implementing new pharmacy IT systems in mental health is complex due to the wide geographical areas covered and the wide range of providers.
- NWW is unlikely to work if the workforce is too small to bring about change.

Working within the multidisciplinary team

Good mental health services usually result from effective teams who are able to incorporate a wide range of professional skills for the benefit of the service user. The participation of pharmacy staff as members of multidisciplinary teams occurs at various levels of the organisation:

- The chief pharmacist, as a member of the senior management team, ensures that systems are in place to support the best use of medicines across organisational and professional boundaries.
- The chief pharmacist's role is to assure the MHT of good medicines governance. For many MHTs, the multidisciplinary committee that supports this role of medicines governance is the DTC.
- The specialist mental health clinical pharmacist, as a member of the ward or community multidisciplinary team, takes leadership for medicines management and has control over the medicines use and responsibility for the dissemination of medicines information.
- The pharmacy technician's role, is as a member of the ward or community team with responsibility for the ordering and supply of medicines for the service and for individual service users who are newly admitted, taking leave or being discharged. The pharmacy technician also has responsibility for the provision of medicines information to service users.
- As a multidisciplinary team member the pharmacy assistant role consists of ensuring an adequate supply of stock medicines on wards and teams, and the generation of routine medicines orders.

Conclusion

Medicines management cannot be achieved by any profession working in isolation; to succeed the process must be led. Currently mental health services are undergoing many changes and the roles of professional groups are developing in light of initiatives brought about by NWW. In the near future, pharmacy services will develop new roles and responsibilities. Colleagues on wards and community teams, in out-patient clinics and specialist services will experience the benefit of increased access to expert skills and knowledge relating to medicines and medicines management.

Increasingly within MHTs the chief pharmacist is responsible for ensuring good medicines management throughout the organisation.

Pharmacists and pharmacy staff in general are an important resource that is available to support nurses and other professionals in their roles within medicines management.

References

Audit Commission (2001) *A Spoonful of Sugar – Medicines Management in NHS Hospitals.* Audit Commission, London.

Boardman, J. & Parsonage, M. (2007) *Delivering the Government's Mental Health Policies – Services, Staffing and Costs.* The Sainsbury Centre for Mental Health, London.

Branford, D., Parton, G., Taylor, D. & Sutton, J. (2006a) *Summary and key findings of the report on the mental health and learning disabilities secondary care pharmacy workforce survey.* National Institute for Mental Health for England, London.

Branford, D., Parton, G., Taylor, D. & Sutton, J. (2006b) *The UKPPG and CMHP report on the mental health and learning disabilities secondary care pharmacy workforce survey (phase 2).* NWW/National Institute for Mental Health For England, London.

Department of Health (1999) *National service framework for mental health: modern standards and service models.* Department of Health, London.

Department of Health (2006) *Improving patients' access to medicines: a guide to implementing nurse and pharmacist independent prescribing within the NHS in England.* Department of Health, London.

Healthcare Commission (2007a) *Talking about medicines. the management of medicines in trusts providing mental health services.* Commission for Healthcare Audit and Inspection, London.

Healthcare Commission (2007b) *The best medicine – the management of medicines in acute and specialist trusts. Acute hospitals portfolio review.* Commission for Healthcare Audit and Inspection, London.

Pratt, P. & Branford, D. (2007) *Learning Lessons from the Spread Programme – Analysis of Key Themes.* NWW/National Institute for Mental Health, London.

Taylor, D.A. & Sutton, J. (2006) *Report on the Mental Health & Learning Disabilities Pharmacy Workforce Survey.* University of Bath, Bath.

Engagement and working collaboratively with service users

Jacquie White and Stuart Wix

Introduction

Engagement and collaboration are key principles which underpin the medicines management process; without these all other interventions are likely to be ineffective. The development of a trusting relationship between the service user and mental health practitioner represents the first phase of any intervention. Building rapport enables both parties to engage in this relationship. It is the most fundamental of all therapeutic strategies and has been described as the 'foundation stone of future work' (Fowler et al., 1998). Mental health literature frequently makes reference to the importance of engagement, particularly in mental health nursing:

> *'Effective nursing is predicated on effective engagement with the person. Only through engaging with the person will the nurse come to understand the nature of the person's needs, and what might need to be offered to address them.'*

> *Cutcliffe & Barker (2002), p. 618*

Engagement does not just refer to the important process of building the therapeutic relationship; it is also about building mutual understanding, confidence and hope for the future. It is important that the service user is involved in the process and that both parties believe that, with their mutual commitment and effort, positive future change can take place (Repper, 2000; MacAllister & Walsh, 2003).

Why is engagement necessary?

Service users often have a range of bio-psychosocial stressors to cope with. These stressors may erode the person's capacity to build trusting relationships and can lead to more widespread isolation, disengagement from services and social exclusion. These stressors include both internal and external factors, for example positive and negative symptoms of psychosis, cognitive deficits, communication difficulties, medication side effects, concurrent alcohol or substance misuse, personality problems, cultural beliefs, history of abuse, stigma and/or racism, homelessness, past medication treatment or services which were perceived by the service user as frightening, painful, degrading or disempowering.

Service users may find it difficult to engage in relationships if their basic needs for safety and survival are not met or they are preoccupied with some other concern. For example, if the service user is having difficulties budgeting for food they are unlikely to prioritise a meeting with their worker that involves a bus journey that they can ill-afford. It may be necessary to work with the service user to address practical concerns, such as benefits issues, before starting the medicines management intervention. Specific medication issues may also need to be addressed early on in the process to maximise the potential for engagement. For example, if the service user has what appears to be many negative symptoms of psychosis and/or extrapyramidal side effects, neuroleptic-induced deficit syndrome may be suspected and a reduction in dose or change to an atypical antipsychotic may be required.

The practitioner needs to engage by taking a holistic view of the person's current problems and needs, in order to better formulate an understanding of the service user's problems. The essential role of the worker is therefore an active one and may include reaching out to the person to attempt to bridge any gap with those around him or her (Kingdon, 1998).

Core skills for developing engagement

There are several core skills required for engaging with service users with serious mental health problems:

- addressing or stabilising external factors which impact on the service user's ability to engage;
- listening to the service user's account of his or her story and perceptions in a positive and empathic manner;
- adopting a flexible and collaborative approach;

- building connections with others;
- taking a long-term perspective;
- maintaining hope and optimism;
- scaling the level of engagement.

Certain conditions are required for the initial building of any helping relationship. These originate in a humanistic philosophy where each individual, whatever their circumstances, is considered to have the potential for growth, change and self-development (Rogers, 1989). The worker's task is to provide the optimal conditions to help the person feel valued, accepted and prepared to trust. Rogers (1989) describes three core conditions of this person centred approach:

- *unconditional positive regard*, which is described as an attitude that offers 'warm acceptance . . . a "prizing" of the person . . . caring for the client . . . as a separate person, with permission to have his own feelings, his own experiences' (p. 225);
- *genuineness*, which he describes as being 'a congruent, genuine, integrated person . . . . . . the opposite of presenting a façade' (p. 224) and
- *empathy*, which is 'to sense the client's private world as if it were your own, but without ever losing the "as if" quality'(p. 226).

These conditions, validating the person and his or her experiences, are all central to the therapeutic communication techniques of active listening.

This interpersonal approach needs to be supplemented with a structured, goal-directed intervention to support the person with serious mental illness to organise him or herself and take action. Time needs to be spent early on to find shared goals, which both parties can sign up to and work towards. If it takes 10 sessions to determine goals then it takes 10 sessions. Flexibility and pragmatism are crucial if engagement and collaboration are to work.

Flexibility and pragmatism

It is important to be flexible regarding where, when and how often to meet to discuss medication. The agenda for the session should be collaboratively agreed at the beginning of each session and the practitioner should check with the service user if there are any other more pressing concerns. This facilitates ownership of the medicines management process by the service user but also allows the work to be adapted to meet different presentations and needs on different days and times. The practitioner should be prepared to focus on more immediate concerns, if required, and postpone the planned agenda for another day or time.

Involving family and friends

Engagement with carers, friends and other health and social care workers can be vitally important, and part of the practitioner's role may be to facilitate or work to repair these relationships. Carers and friends have a wealth of information, which can be harnessed by the service user to understand his or her own medicines management needs and to plan relapse prevention strategies (e.g. when completing a timeline or crisis plan). Including family members and friends in the assessment process is often useful and becomes even more important when the cultural experience of the service user (gender, race, class, experience) is different to that of the practitioner. Beliefs about mental illness, symptoms and medication can all be culturally determined. For example, service users may believe medication should work immediately or have little faith in the practitioner due to their gender or status or both. Symptoms can be incorrectly identified due to cultural differences. It may be necessary to check out any apparent delusional beliefs anonymously with other members of the service user's community, for example voluntary groups (Luthra & Diniesh, 2000).

Carers often report feeling excluded from services due to concerns about confidentiality. By taking a positive stance, stating how it is usual to work with families and friends, and asking the service user who they want to be included from the start is a good way to avoid future problems. Good relationships across the primary and secondary care interface are also important to enable the service user to access timely repeat prescriptions and physical health monitoring. Although the practitioner cannot promote the use of a particular (commercial) community pharmacist, it is often possible to support service users to build relationships with their usual pharmacists so that they can approach them with medication questions and concerns. This may also have the benefit of promoting normalisation, as it is usual to seek medication advice from pharmacists on the high street and pharmacies are often open when other services are closed.

Collaboration

Although the development of an active collaborative relationship is a key aim in medicines management, dilemmas can arise in the relationship. For example, when service users express the desire to discontinue medication, against a history of prolonged or dangerous relapses, practitioners are caught between their concern for the service users exposing themselves to the possibility of a relapse against their role of enabling service users to become central to the decision-making process and the prospect of jeopardising the long-term relationship. However, collaboration requires both parties to work together to help identify and solve problems. Workers should not assume that they know what works best for a person in a particular set of circumstances. Instead the approach to be taken is one of constant learning where both parties explore possible solutions and then use this to help formulate the client's problems and the next steps to be taken.

Practitioners should always consider the circumstances of the individual service users and engage them in a self-assessment of the issues for them; helping the service users to weigh up the benefits and risks of medication, examine their beliefs, problem solve and set realistic and achievable goals for the future. It is the role of the worker to exchange information in an accessible and balanced format; this should include information about the rationale for taking medication, not just side effects. Any anxiety about promoting non-compliance by telling the service user the truth about potential side effects is unfounded. There is plenty of research evidence that education and information-giving interventions do not lead to poor adherence (Gray et al., 2002). There are clear benefits in engaging service users in a dialogue about their medications where they can raise concerns, ask questions and examine their beliefs.

Although it is important to agree specific and realistic goals in the short term, keeping some long-term goals in sight can help to maintain commitment to a process that may seem to be taking a long time. This also helps the service user to associate medicines management with goals which may otherwise appear to be unrelated but whose success may be contingent on preventing relapse, for example obtaining a flat, starting an education course.

Self-awareness

Self-awareness allows workers to make conscious decisions about their choice of verbal and non-verbal communication in the interaction with the service users and is probably the most important skill for effective communication. It is necessary to examine one's own reluctance to engage with ideas and perceptions of the service users or their carers and, in doing this, evaluate the extent of our own resistance to change. Arguing, denying, interrupting or ignoring behaviours are a clue to practitioners that service users are defending themselves against anxiety about change by resisting progress. Practitioners should recognise this as an indication that it is time to stop and re-evaluate the appropriateness of their approach at that time and for that stage of change. Particular care needs to be taken where there are cultural differences between the worker and the service user so that cultural behaviours or perceptions are not misinterpreted as resistant. For example, poor eye contact and gaze aversion may be culturally determined. It is vitally important that the worker avoids being 'hooked' into high-expressed emotion behaviours such as confrontation, criticism or over involvement (Gamble, 2000). Avoiding resistance is an important goal of the medicines management intervention and a clear task of the worker (Gray & Robson, 2004). Self-awareness can be promoted by continually re-evaluating one's own attitudes, beliefs and expressed emotion characteristics through self-reflection and clinical supervision.

Informed choice and medicines management

Information sharing is vital to the development of a positive relationship (Wills, 1982) and can be seen as reducing clients' anxiety and increasing their autonomy. The information given when seeking consent is often sensitive in that it relates to the experience of the service user. It broaches topics such as diagnosis, symptoms and side effects of medication. Often the language used is either new to the service user or has previously been experienced as labelling or stigmatising. This can lead to an increase in anxiety. It is not enough to provide factual information to the service user; it is necessary to establish a relationship where the person feels safe to explore the relevance of the material to his or her individual situation and experience. For service users to gain maximum benefit from the information and understand it from the context of their circumstances, the practitioner needs to revisit the information periodically and indeed prompt service users to review and revise their understanding.

Practice rituals such as requiring the service user to queue for a 'medication round' or attend a large multidisciplinary 'ward round' can mediate against a process of informed choice by increasing anxiety and reducing the opportunity for the service user's voice to be heard or questions asked. It is also unusual for the rationale for prescribed medication to be presented to service users, their carers and even members of the multidisciplinary team. If it is presented it is often in the language of psychiatry rather than that of the service user. For example, it is common to see anticholinergic medication prescribed for the unspecific and abbreviated 'EPSE' (extrapyramidal side effects), or sodium valproate may be prescribed to stabilise mood, to prevent seizures and even to raise the plasma concentration of a concurrent antipsychotic, for example in a heavy smoker. One can see how confusion can arise if the rationale for the prescription is not specifically made from the outset. These rituals and practices have arisen in a healthcare system that is traditionally paternalistic and aims to protect the service user from difficult and potentially distressing information (Harris et al., 2002). One way to try and change this culture is to introduce medicines management care planning, where the specific and individualised rationale for the medication, need for any intervention and agreed collaborative goals, monitoring and frequency of review are documented together with, and importantly in, the language of the service user (White, 2004).

Informed consent

Assessment of the capacity of individuals to take autonomous decisions is essentially a values-based judgement (Fulbrook, 1994; Dimond, 2008). In mental health and learning disability nursing, professional guidelines state that the nurse 'must always work from the assumption that the clients have the capacity to consent' (NMC Archived UKCC Publication, 1998). In practice this often means that a variety of compliant behaviours are interpreted as consent and questions about capacity only arise when the person is actively refusing treatment. This is further complicated by a legal system that does not recognise informed consent outside of common law and holds implied consent as being as equally valid as verbal or written consent (Dimond, 1995). Advance directives have been proposed as a way to allow service users to specify their wishes for future medication treatment should they lose capacity and be deemed unable to make decisions. However, difficulties can arise when trying to incorporate them into current mental health legislation and practice as a prior refusal to accept treatment would probably be accepted for a voluntary patient but could be over-ruled if the person is detained under the *Mental Health Act 1983* (Atkinson et al., 2003). Collaborative crisis and/or medication-focused care plans signed by the service user and the team can prompt information to be provided and future plans for treatment to be specified and negotiated. Such plans may be more empowering and start to change the legacy of the paternalistic culture by engaging professionals in a more equal relationship with service users.

In a grounded theory study into the lived experience of mental health professionals and service users, Barker et al. (1999) identified a 'translation dimension' of mental health nursing. Nurses were valued by service users for 'telling the truth' about medication rather than 'what the doctor wanted them to hear'. This suggests nurses may be considering alternative views within the therapeutic relationship. One of the roles of the nurse was seen by both other mental health team professionals and service users as 'a "go between", bridging the lay world of the person and family, and the professional world of the psychiatric team' (p. 280).

To achieve the roles of 'translator' and 'go between', while respecting the autonomy of the service user, is a tall order. In medicines management, as with any intervention, it is necessary to use a variety of assessments to evaluate ongoing needs, and monitor risk and progress. To achieve this, the subjective experience and observed behaviour of the person is labelled, recorded and categorised within a particular classification system and timeframe. This task involves the practitioner interpreting the service user's experiences in objective terms. However, to ensure consent to treatment is informed, the practitioner must translate the jargon of psychiatry into language that the service users can understand, engage with and use to enter a dialogue to explore what their medication means to them and take an active part in the treatment process. To achieve this role in particular, the practitioner must step outside the scientific mind-set and consider the meaning of medication to the person, from their individual point of view and experience, without prejudice. This sort of relating is informed by a humanistic-existential paradigm and uses phenomenological (qualitative) methods. One way of dealing with this dilemma in the authors' experience is to develop a flexibility to alternate between ways of relating and thinking in practice, depending on the needs of the service user at the time. This is a complex and difficult task, requiring a broad knowledge base of several paradigms, an ability to communicate in the language of psychiatry and the service user, an ability to apply these when appropriate in different situations and a developed sense of self-awareness. The role the practitioner adopts during the medicines management process is based on the needs of the service user at any given moment. A model proposed by Usher & Arthur (1997, 1998) is useful here as it recognises the need to adopt different roles in different phases of the relationship and in different circumstances. Particular roles (based on work by Peplau[1]) are adopted to match need along a continuum from advocacy to empowerment while maintaining issues of power in the forefront of decision-making.

At the beginning of the relationship, the practitioner is in the role of stranger and encourages the service user to engage in the intervention. This is also the time to address the boundaries of the relationship, agree mutual goals and agendas, and sort out the practical issues of where and when to meet and when the sessions will end. Although collaboration here is the goal it may sometimes be necessary to adopt a surrogate (paternalistic) role, and advocate needs *for* the service user, for example

[1] In her psychodynamic theory of nursing Peplau (1952) described four phases, orientation, exploitation, working and resolution, and six roles in the nurse–patient relationship: stranger, surrogate, counsellor, leader, resource person and teacher.

if the service user is experiencing debilitating side effects or has problems which impair communication or assert preferences. In the working phase of the intervention a more active partnership is developed; supporting the service user to gain and practise skills in problem solving and expressing his or her own medicines management needs to others. This can involve adopting both a leadership and counselling role. The role of teacher may be appropriate to any of these phases, for example providing information about the rationale for and benefits and risks of medication. However, the aim of medicines management is to enable service users to become self-efficacious at managing their treatment and in this context the objective is to support service users to find this information out for themselves by signposting rather than didactically instructing. As they develop the skill, knowledge and understanding in managing all aspects of their pharmacological treatment, the time spent working on medicines management issues reduces. Some of the issues are explored in the case study given in Box 9.1.

Box 9.1 Case study

The following case study is of a 28-year-old single man with a 10-year history of schizophrenia and a coexisting substance use. He has been prescribed various antipsychotic medications over the years with limited effect and is currently prescribed an oral antipsychotic. He has only partially responded to this drug and continues to complain of auditory hallucinations and a significant gain in weight. Additionally he has complained about sexual dysfunction, and he has indicated to his community psychiatric nurse (CPN) that he is contemplating stopping taking his oral antipsychotic medication in the future.

Engagement

The community mental health team have been responsible for this service user's care for the past 5 years and have found it increasingly difficult to engage him in discussing his medication and his past history of non-adherence with oral antipsychotic treatment. As a strategy for improved future engagement, and to reduce his resistance to talking about medication, the team elected to withdraw from talking about medication in the short term and focus more upon other aspects of his care by helping him to address his accommodation and benefit needs. In helping him sort out aspects of his social care, the team were then able to return in a graduated way to more focused discussion regarding the subject of taking medication. The team introduced more structure to each session and a collaborative agenda was agreed for each session.

Summary of assessment

The service user was prescribed a newer antipsychotic to be taken by orally twice a day. He obtained his medication from a local pharmacy where he would take his prescription every 4 weeks, following a regular monthly appointment with his CPN, who was a registered independent prescriber. The service user indicated that he occasionally forgot to collect his prescription, which resulted in an inconsistent pattern of taking his medication. As a consequence, his symptoms were poorly controlled and he was particularly distressed by his voices, which would criticise him constantly. He claimed that in order to mitigate the distress he experienced as result of the voices he would habitually smoke two or more joints of cannabis on a daily basis, which helped him to relax. The service user was concerned that he was experiencing sexual dysfunction since he had commenced the oral antipsychotic, which was having an adverse impact on his relationship with his girlfriend.

Medicines management interventions

The service user was given an opportunity to reflect back upon his experiences of taking treatment, and was invited to talk about the negative aspects in detail, starting at any point in the past that he believed to be significant in his life. He described his experiences at school from the age of 16, where he had few friends, felt isolated and took solace in drinking large quantities of cider. By the age of 18 years, he described hearing whispering coming from his wardrobe, which he attributed to 'evil spirits' and became so frightened by the experience on one occasion that he barricaded himself in his bedroom. His mother became very concerned and subsequently called the police, who took him to a police station where he had his first contact with a psychiatrist. This then led to his first admission to hospital for assessment and treatment, which lasted 12 weeks. He described the experience as frightening, as he was wary of staff and other patients. During the early part of his admission he was restrained by staff and was given an injection that made him feel very drowsy and lethargic. He was later offered an oral antipsychotic, which he took whilst in hospital, and noticed that the experience of 'evil spirits' (auditory hallucinations) declined. However, he felt sluggish and experienced a tremor of both hands when he took the medication. He was discharged on oral medication and over a period of time took his medication less frequently. He has been admitted to hospital on four occasions in the past 5 years under similar circumstances. He has been under the care of a continuing care team in the community for the last 5 years, receives regular visits from the CPN and attends the outpatient department on a monthly basis to be reviewed by his psychiatrist.

Continued

His latest discussion with his psychiatrist and CPN has revealed that his erratic pattern of taking oral medication has resulted from his ongoing concerns about its side effects and a lack of a shared perspective on his part. His medication was reviewed by the CPN, with the side effects he had described taken into consideration, and he was prescribed an alternative atypical antipsychotic, which is not known to cause sexual dysfunction and is less sedating.

Exploring ambivalence

The service user was ambivalent about taking medication as he was uncertain as to whether it had a direct effect upon his experiences of hearing voices. It was explained to the service user that it is common and normal to be uncertain about taking medication. He was offered the opportunity to talk about the not-so-good and the good things about taking medication.

Beliefs about medication

The service user was 80% certain that he did not need medication. He also believed that smoking cannabis helped him with the voices, helped him relax, yet acknowledged that, after a sustained period of use, it made him feel increasingly paranoid. He agreed to monitor his voices over the course of a week and rate how distressed he was by them. He was also asked to record each time he took his medication and smoked cannabis. When he was asked to rate himself again about his belief that he did not need to take medication (once he felt better), his rating changed from 80% to 40%, indicating a more positive perception of the value of medication.

Looking forward

The service user wanted to venture out more from his flat and enrolled at a local college, with the support of his social worker and CPN, to undertake an access course. He recognised that when he stopped taking medication he was more suspicious of others, was increasingly fearful of his surroundings and was less likely to venture out of his flat. Learning from the past enabled him to set up a support system to assist him to remain at college and avoid slipping back into previous coping behaviours, such as smoking cannabis. This also included being more organised about collecting his prescription from the chemist.

Conclusion

At the practice level, the skills needed to communicate with service users about their medication appear very complex. Practitioners must be able to understand the scientific treatment view and be able to critically evaluate its evidence base. They must also be able to develop understanding of the health beliefs and views of the service user. The practitioner needs to be up-to-date in both the biological paradigm and cultural and lay beliefs of mental health. There is a need for the practitioner to be able to communicate freely in both the language of psychiatry and in the language of the service user and move with ease between the two. Relationship, assertiveness and liaison skills are needed to build lines of communication to facilitate support for the service user's decision-making in the wider system. In all, communication about treatment and issues of power must be kept at the forefront of self-awareness to avoid coercion in the interaction. Because of the complexity of this task, there is an urgent need for effective supervision, ongoing education and support of this role in practice.

References

Atkinson, J.M., Garner, H.C., Patrick, H. & Stuart, S. (2003) Issues in the development of advance directives in mental health care. *Journal of Mental Health*, **12**(5), 463–474.

Barker, P., Jackson, S. & Stevenson, C. (1999) What are psychiatric nurses needed for? Developing a theory of essential nursing practice. *Journal of Psychiatric and Mental Health Nursing*, **6**, 273–282.

Cutcliffe, J.R. & Barker, P. (2002) Considering the care of the suicidal client and the case for 'engagement and inspiring hope' or 'observations'. *Journal of Psychiatric and Mental Health Nursing*, **9**, 611–621.

Dimond, B. (1995) *Legal Aspects of Nursing*. 2nd edn. Prentice Hall, London.

Dimond, B. (2008) *Legal Aspects of Mental Capacity*. Wiley-Blackwell, Oxford.

Fowler, D., Garety, P. & Kuipers, L. (1998) Cognitive therapy for psychosis: formulation, treatment effects and service implications. *Journal of Mental Health*, **7**, 123–133.

Fulbrook, P. (1994) Assessing mental competence of patients and relatives. *Journal of Advanced Nursing*, **20**, 457–461.

Gamble, C. (2000) Using a low expressed emotion approach to develop positive therapeutic alliances. In: Gamble, C. & Brennan, G. (eds) *Working with Serious Mental Illness: A Manual for Clinical Practice*. Baillière Tindall, London.

Gray, R. & Robson, D. (2004) *Concordance Skills: Collaboration, Involvement, Choice: A Manual for Mental Health Workers*. Institute of Psychiatry, Kings College, London.

Gray, R., Wykes, T. & Gournay, K. (2002) From compliance to concordance: A review of the literature to enhance compliance with antipsychotic medication. *Journal of Psychiatric and Mental Health Nursing*, **9**, 277–284.

Harris, N., Lovell, K. & Day, J. (2002) Consent and long-term neuroleptic treatment. *Journal of Psychiatric and Mental Health Nursing*, **9**, 475–482.

Kingdon, D. (1998) Cognitive behavioural therapy of psychosis: Complexities in engagement and therapy. In: Tarrier, N., Wells, A. & Haddock, G. (eds) *Treating Complex Cases: The Cognitive Behavioural Therapy Approach*. Bailliere Tindall. Elsevier Ltd., Edinburgh.

Luthra, A. & Diniesh, B. (2000) Serious mental illness: cross cultural issues. In: Gamble, C. & Brennan, G. (eds) *Working With Serious Mental Illness: A Manual for Clinical Practice*. Harcourt., London.

MacAllister, M. & Walsh, K. (2003) CARE: A framework for mental health practice. *Journal of Psychiatric and Mental Health Nursing*, **10**, 39–48.

NMC Archived UKCC Publication (1998) *UKCC guidelines for mental health and learning disability nursing NMC* [online] UK. Available at www.nmc-uk.org/aFrameDisplay.aspx?DocumentID=521&Keyword= (accessed 29 May 2008).

Peplau, H.E. (1952) *Interpersonal Relations in Nursing*. G.P. Putnam's Sons, New York.

Repper, J. (2000) The helping relationship. In: Harris, N., Williams, S. & Bradshaw, T. (eds) *Psychosocial Interventions for People with Schizophrenia: A Practical Guide for Mental Health Workers*. Palgrave Macmillan, Basingstoke.

Rogers, C.R. (1989) A theory of therapy, personality, and interpersonal relationships as developed in the client-centered framework. In: Kirschenbaum, H. & Henderson, V. L. (eds) *The Carl Rogers Reader*. Houghton Mifflin, Boston.

Usher, K. & Arthur, D. (1997) Nurses and neuroleptic medication; applying theory to a working relationship with clients and their families. *Journal of Psychiatric and Mental Health Nursing*, **4**, 117–123.

Usher, K. & Arthur, D. (1998) Process consent: a model for enhancing informed consent in mental health nursing. *Journal of Advanced Nursing*, **27**, 692–697.

White, J. (2004) Medication management. In: Ryan, T. & Pritchard, J. (eds) *Good Practice in Adult Mental Health*. Jessica Kingsley, London.

Wills, T.A. (1982) *Basic Processes in Helping Relationships*. Academic Press, New York.

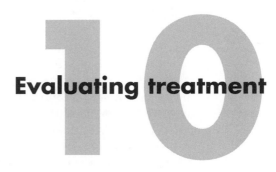

Evaluating treatment

Jennie Day and Neil Harris

Introduction

Psychotropic medications have an individualistic response for the people who take them. A person's subjective experience of medication effects is idiosyncratic; the same dose of the same drug can be taken by three people, with complete symptom relief and no problems for one person, distressing side effects and no symptom relief for the second, and no effect for the third. Because of this, it is important to take an individualised approach when evaluating treatment. To assist in this process we will describe the assessment tools available for assessing symptoms and response, side effects of treatment, and attitudes to treatment.

In this era of evidence-based guidelines it is easy to overlook the evidence we can gather from individuals. A meta-analysis of the information gained from a number of research studies will provide evidence of treatment efficacy for the majority of people but it does not help decide which treatment will best suit an individual. This is the same for the range of psychotropic medications prescribed for psychological difficulties. The treatment of schizophrenia provides a good example of the need for an individualised approach. Seventy per cent of people with a diagnosis of schizophrenia may benefit from a particular antipsychotic but if you are not one of those 70% this evidence is irrelevant. In addition, only one-third of people prescribed antipsychotics will have a complete remission of symptoms, a third will show only amelioration of symptoms. The National Institute of Clinical Excellence (NICE) (2002) guidelines recommend atypical antipsychotics for first-line treatment of newly diagnosed schizophrenia, but some people have an excellent response from a conventional antipsychotic with minimal side effects, whereas atypical antipsychotics can cause unendurable side effects or a lack of efficacy for some people. For an individual, the choice to take treatment can be a complex analysis of the relative costs and benefits of treatment and the impact of the treatment on everyday life, as well as individual health beliefs. This may explain why recent research has indicated that there is little difference between first- and second-generation antipsychotics in terms of quality of life (Jones et al., 2006).

Assessments can help us to build a picture of aspects of a person's response to treatment, including symptoms, side effects and contraindications of treatment, attitudes to treatment and the impact of treatment on day-to-day domestic, vocational and recreational life. However, the most important thing about assessment is doing something constructive with the information. Too many assessments lay dormant and unscored in dusty case notes and, needless to say, this is not good practice. This chapter will explore the methods that can be used to assess a person's mental health and treatment and outline practical methods to aid medication management in mental health.

There is an increasing emphasis on a model of shared decision-making with the service user at the centre of treatment decisions. The National Health Service Plan (Department of Health, 2005) outlined that healthcare workers should:

- respect people for their knowledge and understanding of their own experience, their own clinical condition, their experience of the illness and how it impacts on their life;
- provide people with the information and choices that allow them to feel in control;
- ensure everyone receives not just high-quality clinical care but care with consideration for their needs at all times;
- treat people as human beings and as individuals, not just people to be processed;
- ensure people always feel valued by the health service and are treated with respect, dignity and compassion;
- understand that the best judges of their experience are the people themselves;
- ensure that mental health care is available to people in the most trouble-free way, minimising disruption to their life;
- explain what happens if things go wrong and why, and agree the way forward.

Informal assessment

To begin this chapter we will look at the importance of making informal observations and initiating discussions that may prompt the use of standardised assessment tools to gain more detail or indicate areas that need to be addressed. There will be many factors that contribute to the health of a person and the effectiveness of medication. It is important to be mindful of how the person's current and changing circumstances can affect how the medication is working. Discussions about these factors can help identify things that are impeding health and the effectiveness of medication. When a compromise to health is discovered a dialogue can take place about the action that needs to be taken.

Through time people change the way they live life. The lifestyle changes that people adopt through engaging in new opportunities or responding to negative life events can have effects on how medicines are metabolised or exposure to additional side effects. Engaging with a 'stop smoking' programme is a positive action both physically and psychologically. Yet if the person is taking a psychotropic medication this action may result in toxicity or adverse reactions as the metabolism of the drug is slowed down as liver enzymes return to normal. For a person who starts to drink alcohol or increases their intake, as a result of a personal misfortune, further complications can arise. The combination of psychotropic medicines and alcohol can accumulate their individual effects, further depressing the central nervous system (CNS). This can result in toxic levels and enhances the effects of intoxication: sedation, poor co-ordination, judgement and concentration.

Ongoing discussions about physical health can reveal ailments that can, for example, affect mood or may be indicated as a risk factor for serious conditions such as neuroleptic malignant syndrome. Other, minor conditions can prompt the person to get an over-the-counter remedy, but this can be problematic. For example, the use of antacids can reduce the serum level of some antipsychotics whereas antibiotics can increase the serum level of lithium.

Caffeine intake of between 600 and 750 mg per day is considered excessive with 1000 mg well into the toxic range. These levels of toxicity may result from the consumption of as few as six or seven mugs of instant coffee, and a bit more for tea. In addition, caffeine can be found in cola, milk chocolate, energy drinks and analgesics. The adverse effects of high levels of caffeine include insomnia, anxiety, restlessness, tension, irritability, auditory and visual hallucinations. It can cause tremor, muscle twitching and poor concentration. For people with mental health problems some of their symptoms, which may be considered as part of the illness or side effects of medication, may be because of excessive consumption of drinks containing caffeine. It is therefore an important area of enquiry when conducting assessments. Enabling a reduction of excessive caffeine intake can have dramatic results in improving thinking processes and a person's mental health in general. However, caffeine reduction can be difficult to achieve and people found to be dependent can suffer withdrawal symptoms, such as headaches, sedation, depression, fatigue and lethargy (Bazaire, 2007).

Agreement that it may be causing a difficulty, identifying an acceptable alternative drink and slow substitution are useful ways forward. Monitoring for positive effects is an important reinforcer for continued abstinence.

Why use assessment measures?

Health professionals do not routinely ask or know what symptoms or side effects a service user experiences. It has been found that health professionals overestimate the benefits and underestimate the adverse effects of medical treatment (Horne et al., 2001a). Repeated studies have found that service users consistently complain about a lack of information given to them about medication, particularly side effects, and if someone does not know that a condition is a side effect he or she may not report it. In the Healthcare Commission (2007) survey of 6169 users of mental health services it was found that 8% were not told the purpose of mental health medication and that 33% had not had side effects of medication explained. Many service users do not routinely ask or volunteer information, and so it is important for health professionals to assess all service users in a similar way so that they receive equitable treatment.

Assessments can provide an objective measure of an attribute, whereas clinical impression, which is often used in clinical practice, has poor reliability and validity. It is important that an assessment tool has good validity (that is, that the assessment actually measures what it is designed to measure) and reliability (the characteristic of a measurement tool to produce consistent results, over time, on two or more occasions to the same subject) in the population in which it is used. As well as being valid and reliable it is important that an assessment tool used in clinical practice is practical in terms of the time taken to administer it, the ease of scoring and interpretation of scores. In this chapter we have attempted to indicate those assessment tools that are of practical value.

The other benefit of carrying out formal assessments is that it provides lasting information that can be stored in case notes and referred back to. Thus, when staff change there is a formal record of, for example, response to a particular medication. It would be ideal if the assessments of medication, including response, side effects and attitudes to treatment, could be summarised so that they could be referred to at a glance to aid future prescribing decisions. Unfortunately, this is often not the case and it is hoped that in the new age of electronic records and prescribing in the NHS, recording summaries of prescribed medication and related assessments would become routine practice, making them easily accessible to all relevant health practitioners.

It is important that there is a good therapeutic alliance between the service user and the health practitioner as this will provide more accurate assessments, and improved agreement between staff and service users leads to improved clinical outcomes (Gabbay et al., 2003; Junghan et al., 2007; Lasalvia, 2008). Studies consistently show that healthcare workers and service users have divergent opinions on mental healthcare needs and treatment options. Health service workers tend to be more focused on diagnosis and treatment, whilst service users tend to be more focused on problems related to social integration. In this sense, practitioners emphasise the elimination of symptoms whereas the focus for service users is recovery, and practitioners need to be mindful that their priorities may be in conflict with those of the person they are working with.

Key measures

Symptoms

Psychotropic medications are prescribed to eliminate or reduce symptoms of mental illness, therefore the primary way of estimating the efficacy of a medication regimen is to undertake assessments of psychiatric symptoms. As with the assessment of medication side effects, global assessments of mental state, undertaken on a regular basis, can highlight the need to complete more targeted assessment tools seeking more detail and better understanding. It is important to bear in mind that response to psychotropic medication varies widely. For example, with antipsychotics one-third of people with a diagnosis of schizophrenia respond well with significant symptom reduction, approximately one-third of people respond partially and 20–30% have no response at all to antipsychotics. An adequate trial of an antipsychotic would be 6 weeks so it would make sense to measure symptoms at baseline and then 6 weeks after changing/initiating a drug or changing the dose.

The following describes an assessment pathway for a person diagnosed as suffering from a psychotic disorder. The assessments described here are commonly seen in practice. Alternative assessments are available which may be suited to particular circumstances and new assessments, with improved psychometric properties, are frequently available in academic journals.

The Kraweika, Goldberg and Vaughn or
Psychiatric Assessment Scale

A commonly used measure for undertaking a global psychopathology assessment is the KGV (Kraweika et al., 1977) or Psychiatric

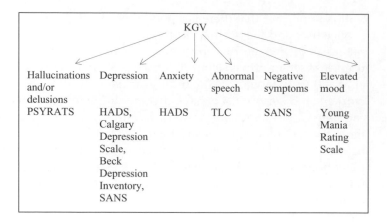

Figure 10.1 Filtering global psychopathological assessment to detailed assessments.

Assessment Scale (PAS), modified by Lancashire (University of Manchester). This comprehensive assessment consists of 14 dimensions; six from the interview and focus on anxiety, depression, suicidal ideation, elevated mood, delusions and hallucinations. Seven areas of observation include flattened affect, incongruous affect, overactivity, psychomotor retardation, abnormal speech, poverty of speech and abnormal movements. A final section considers the accuracy of the interview. The information gathered during this assessment can combine to make a picture of the person's current mental state. Problem areas identified here can prompt further assessment to develop a more comprehensive evaluation of particular symptoms (Figure 10.1).

The Psychotic Symptom Rating Scale
The Psychotic Symptom Rating Scale (PSYRATS) (Haddock et al., 1999) measures the severity and different dimensions of auditory hallucinations and delusions. The hallucinations rating scale seeks information about when they occur, their location, volume and origin, content, the distress and disruption to the person's life they cause and the level of control the person has over them. For delusions, the scale asks questions about how much the belief occupies their thoughts and disrupts their life, how convinced they are that the belief is true and the distress caused. Hallucinations and delusions are primary targets of antipsychotic treatment; detailed information about these symptoms can track people's changing experience, as they recover or deteriorate, informing the prescribing decisions.

The Calgary Depression Scale
The assessment of depression in psychosis can present a difficult clinical picture as depressive symptoms overlap with negative symptoms

and extrapyramidal side effects, and failure to correctly identify the cause could result in an inappropriate prescription of antidepressants. The Calgary Depression Scale (Addington et al., 1993) has been designed to measure the symptoms of depression in people suffering from schizophrenia, eliminating those symptoms that could be a product of the other conditions. Further information to disentangle this group of conditions can be gained by using the rating scale for extrapyramidal symptoms (Simpson & Angus, 1970).

The Hospital Depression and Anxiety Scale

A frequently used assessment, the Hospital Depression and Anxiety Scale (HADS) (Zigmond & Snaith, 1983), is a quick self-rating scale, which can be used when frequent assessment is required, to follow symptoms between global assessment or following medication changes. It can be completed by the person in his or her own time between meetings. It may also be useful in differentiating anxiety from akathisia, where a person's agitated behaviour can be misinterpreted.

Young's Mania Rating Scale

Young's Mania Rating Scale is an 11-item measure of the core symptoms of mania, which include elevated mood, increased activity, less need for sleep, more energy, pressured speech, grandiosity, racing thoughts, overt anger, poor judgement and lack of insight (Young et al., 1978).

The Scale for the Assessment of Thought, Language and Communication

The assessment of thought disorder and negative symptoms is difficult. The Scale for the Assessment of Thought, Language and Communication (TLC) (Andreasen, 1986) is an extensive assessment and provides details (and examples) of 20 types of thought disorder. Similarly, the Scale for the Assessment of Negative Symptoms (SANS) (Andreasen, 1989) gives detail of 30 signs and symptoms across five dimensions. The detail and length of these assessments render them impractical for routine use in most clinical situations but they are useful reference information in specific cases.

Training is required to undertake all these assessments and some, for example the KGV, require substantial training input before being deemed a reliable assessor. A person's specific symptom profile can be identified during the course of assessment and can be used to develop monitoring programmes and symptom diaries. These can be used by service users, as part of a package of medication management, observing for variation in symptoms in response to medication and lifestyle changes.

Side effects

It is widely recommended that service users should undergo comprehensive health checks before initiating antipsychotic treatment, side effects should be regularly monitored during treatment and individuals switched to an alternative treatment if side effects are serious or persistent (Lader, 1999). Unfortunately, routine monitoring of side effects is not always carried out in clinical practice. There are a number of validated scales available for monitoring the side effects of psychotropic drugs. The choice of scale depends on the drug prescribed and the type of side effects to be measured. In clinical practice, many clinicians depend on the service user self-reporting side effects, but research has shown that many patients do not report side effects. When the occurrence of service users spontaneously stating their experience of side effects and the Udvalg for Kliniske Undersogelser (UKU) scale were compared, significantly more side effects were identified using the validated scale (Gruwez et al., 2004). In the past, some clinicians were worried that discussing side effects would make service users highly suggestible and invent side effects. There were also concerns that discussing side effects would cause undue distress and reduce adherence. There is now a substantial amount of evidence that a lack of information causes poor satisfaction with treatment and distress. Research evidence indicates that informing people about their medication including potential side effects does not increase distress or reduce adherence (Macpherson et al., 1996; Chaplin & Kent, 1998; Haw et al., 2001). In addition, service users want to be warned of side effects before they occur and not afterwards.

The most comprehensive and well-validated scale is the UKU scale (Lingjaerde et al., 1987). The UKU scale has been validated with thousands of people prescribed psychotropic medication and is comprehensive, covering psychic, autonomic, hormonal and allergic side effects, weight gain and extrapyramidal side effects. The scale consists of 48 items rated from 0 to 3. The UKU scale also includes a rating of the likely causal relationship between the side effect and the medication. The scale has good reliability and validity and has been used in longitudinal assessments of side effects. However, this scale is intended to be administered by a trained physician and can take up to an hour to carry out.

Table 10.1 lists the main measures that are available to assess side effects of antipsychotic medication. In the past the Simpson and Angus Scale (SAS), which assesses extrapyramidal side effects, and the Abnormal Involuntary Movement Scale (AIMS) which assesses dyskinesias, were widely used. The SAS was developed in the late 1960s and consists of 10 extrapyramidal side effects (EPSEs) on a five-point Likert scale from 0 to 4. There is some evidence for the validity and reliability of the scale. For example, Janno et al. (2005) found the

Table 10.1 Assessment tools for antipsychotic side effects

Author	Year	Type of side effects	Number of items
Simpson & Angus	1970	EPSE	10
NIMH AIMS	1980	Dyskinesia	12
Lingjaerde UKU	1987	All	48
Barnes Barnes Akathisia Rating Scale	1989	Akathisia	4
Sachdev Prince Henry Hospital Akathisia Rating Scale	1994	Akathisia	10
Day et al. LUNSERS	1995	All	41 + 10 red herrings
Yusufi et al. ANNSERS	2005	All	35
Waddell & Taylor	2008	Selected side effects	22

EPSE, extrapyramidal side effects; NIMH, National Institute of Mental Health; AIMS, Abnormal Involuntary Movements Scale; UKU, Udvalg for Kliniske of UndersØgelser (Scandinavian Society of Psychopharmacology Committee of Clinical Investigations).

internal reliability assessed by Cronbach's alpha to be 0.79, and the scale discriminated between people diagnosed with neuroleptic-induced Parkinsonism according to the *Diagnostic and Statistical Manual of Mental Disorders* (4th edn) (DSM IV) criteria. The SAS does not measure bradykinesia or subjective experience of rigidity.

The AIMS scale is a 12-item scale that measures dyskinesias (involuntary movements) of the face and body (Guy, 1976). It also rates incapacitation associated with, and a person's awareness of, dyskinesias. Munetz & Benjamin (1988) give guidance on the practical use of the scale in the clinical setting. It is routinely used to screen for tardive dyskinesias (TDs) and is the most comprehensive scale available for this.

The last two scales have been used in research for many years; they include physical manipulation of the service user and are rather narrow as they focus only on EPSEs. It is difficult to see how these assessments reflect patients' overall experience of adverse effects. For example, the SAS includes the 'head dropping test' and the 'glabella tap', which involves tapping the person's forehead and counting the number of times they blink. It is surprising, given that it is now well documented that atypical antipsychotics are associated with a lower incidence of EPSEs, that these rating scales are still used in clinical trials. It is also noteworthy that the initial trials of atypical antipsychotics used these scales and haloperidol as a comparator, when there is substantial evidence that haloperidol is associated with the highest incidence of EPSEs compared to other antipsychotics. It is important to remember that atypical antipsychotics have their own problems, for example weight gain and effects on glucose metabolism, and that they can still induce EPSEs (particularly at higher doses).

Barnes (1989) developed and validated a scale assessing the severity of akathisia that included subscales of psychological and motor restlessness. The scale consists of four subscales: objective rating (rated 0–3), subjective awareness of restlessness (rated 0–3), subjective distress related to restlessness (rated 0–3) and global clinical assessment of akathisia (rated 0–5). The scale has good reliability and validity and is used widely in research and clinical practice (Barnes, 2003).

The Prince Henry Hospital Akathisia Rating Scale is also a validated tool for the assessment of akathisia. It shows good reliability and validity, including concurrent validity with the Barnes Akathisia Rating Scale (Sachdev, 1994).

The Liverpool University Neuroleptic Side Effects Rating Scale (LUNSERS) is based on the UKU, but is self-administered by the service user and therefore can be carried out in approximately 5–20 minutes. It consists of 41 known side effect items and 10 'red herring' items that were included during the initial validation of the self-rated status of the scale. The side effects are split into six main subgroups of side effects: extrapyramidal, antimuscarinic, hormonal, cardiovascular, allergic and miscellaneous. The items are scored on a Likert scale from 0 to 4, and two items are relevant to females only. The LUNSERS has good reliability and validity. It has good concurrent validity (i.e. where an assessment correlates well with a previously validated assessment measuring the same thing) with the UKU, and a recent study has shown that scores on relevant subscales of the LUNSERS correlate with the Barnes Akathisia Rating Scale and the SAS (Jung et al., 2005). During validation of the LUNSERS, people were prescribed a variety of antipsychotic medication, including atypical antipsychotics, and thus it is valid to use in people prescribed atypical antipsychotics.

Yusufi et al. (2005) reported the development of the Antipsychotic Non-Neurological Side Effect Rating Scale (ANNSERS). The scale looks at collecting a range of information about side effects and treatment complications. It develops a side-effect profile by collecting data by talking to the person, examining case notes and undertaking tests, such as for liver function tests, dyscrasias and electrocardiograms (ECGs). A total of 35 areas of concern are rated by a clinician on a four-point scale – absent, mild, moderate and severe.

Recently a new side-effect scale has been developed, the Glasgow Antipsychotic Side Effect Scale (Wadell & Taylor, 2008), which includes

22 side effects. The items in this scale were selected on the basis of the medical importance of side effects as rated by the authors of the scale and its acceptability as rated by a focus group of service users. The scale is cited as a scale for measuring side effects of second generation antipsychotics but all of the items are included in LUNSERS and there was a high correlation between scores on the two scales. The wording is active, e.g. 'I felt sleepy during the day' and the respondent rates each item as 'never', 'once', 'a few times' or 'every day'. The wording is stated to be simplified compared to LUNSERS and it is shorter, although this means that some side effects are not included. It is not possible for health workers to predict what side effects cause distress so comprehensive assessment of side effects and the distress caused by them is imperative.

In addition to rating scales it is important to monitor changes to a person's physical health, which can be adversely affected by mental health medications. The most prevalent side effect in this category, particularly with atypical antipsychotics, is weight gain. In a recent review Rege (2008) recommends the following three main principles for achieving an optimal trade-off between effectiveness and side effects of antipsychotics:

1. A shared decision-making model between the patient, clinician and carer when choosing an antipsychotic.
2. A commitment to baseline and follow-up monitoring with explicit identification of the responsible individual or team.
3. The adoption of clear structured protocols for clinicians to follow in the case of clinically significant weight gain and metabolic issues, which should incorporate greater collaboration between various health professionals from psychiatric and medical special-ist services.

These principles could apply to monitoring of any adverse effects of antipsychotics and it is obvious that to assess the effects of antipsychot-ics, baseline measurements should be taken, for example weight should be measured before treatment with an antipsychotic begins and then periodically. Assessment is not enough; action must be taken to reduce adverse effects and the distress caused by them.

Evaluating physical health

A review by Penedoa and Dahn (2005) indicated the positive link between physical activity and quality of life, and physical and mental health. For example, it has been shown that physical exercise has ben-eficial effects on mood, reducing symptoms of depression and anxiety, enhancing the feeling of wellbeing and engagement in recovery. People suffering from a serious mental illness are at a higher risk of suffering from a range of physical illnesses. For example, people diagnosed as suffering from schizophrenia are very likely to have a coexisting physical condition, such as cardiovascular disease, diabetes, metabolic syndrome and sexual side effects (Mitchell & Malone, 2006).

Psychotropic medications are implicated in the development of physical health problems. Some of the adverse effects of these medications are both common and serious. They can include excess weight gain, abnormal cardiac arrythmias and increased cardiovascular risk. The mechanism which regulates the use of lipids becomes impaired. Lipids are organic compounds, fats, oils, waxes, sterols and triglycerides, which together with carbohydrates and proteins form the key structural material of living cells. Metabolic syndrome is a cluster of factors that increases the risk for the person to develop heart disease, diabetes and stroke. In this context the prescribing practice of polypharmacy, prescribing more than one antipsychotic medication at the same time, increases the risk of cardiac arrhythmias and sudden death (Waddington et al., 1998) and should only be undertaken after serious consideration and the relevant physical health assessments.

People with mental health problems are likely to receive unsatisfactory physical health care (Department of Health, 2006). A study to examine the equity of physical health care for people diagnosed with schizophrenia and the general population concluded that people with schizophrenia were less likely to receive essential health examinations, blood pressure, cholesterol levels or enquiries made about smoking status (Roberts et al., 2007). Similarly, it has been found that over half of those diagnosed with schizophrenia (28%, $n = 93$) received inadequate levels of physical checks, including dental and eye tests. This group of people experienced a lower quality of life and more symptoms that reduce cognitive and social functioning. They are less likely to be in paid employment and more likely to misuse alcohol or drugs (Mackell et al., 2005). The physical health needs of people with serious mental illness are likely to go unrecognised, unnoticed and poorly treated (Phelan et al., 2001).

An assumption is often made that people with mental health problems will not attend appointments for health examinations and advice, but this is not the case: people welcome these kinds of interventions. Positive, general and specific health improvement occurs as a result of improved access to primary care (Osborn et al., 2003). In this context, care coordinators, key workers and named nurses are in a strong position to undertake or initiate physical health screening and access to health promotion advice and activities. They can take an important role in enabling access to basic physical health assessment and care from

---

Box 10.1   Constituents of an annual health screen

The Department of Health (2006) has outlined the constituents of a health screen. The annual physical health screening should include:

- demographic details, personal and family history;
- current medication and medication history, including preparations for other conditions, and side-effect assessment or contraindications;
- basic health checks, including blood pressure, pulse and body mass index;
- blood tests and urinalysis;
- lifestyle assessments, including a review of diet, physical activity, smoking, alcohol and use of illicit substances.

their general practitioner (GP). The constituents of an annual health screen are shown in Box 10.1.

Service users, care co-ordinators and named nurses can also use more specialist resources for assistance in this area. For example, in many mental health trusts, specialist services are being developed to address the physical health needs of service users who receive secondary mental health services. The services can have a number of aims:

- to undertake comprehensive physical health screening/examination for those people who do not attend GP practices:
    - those who find it difficult to attend practices because of communication difficulties, long waiting times or feelings of stigma
    - people who are homeless or with chaotic lifestyles, perhaps working with assertive outreach teams (AOT)
    - additionally, within this process, staff can make referrals to health advisors and provide access to other sources of healthy living opportunities and specialist chronic disease management services
- to develop partnerships between secondary and primary services, establishing care and referral pathways, and providing training and support;
- developing, maintaining and supporting partnerships with the public health departments;
- developing a network of health advisory services, dietary advice, smoking cessation and creating increased opportunities for healthy living activities, exercise trainers, walking clubs and leisure centre programmes;
- providing education to the mental health workforce – developing understanding, knowledge and skills to enable focused work with service users on physical health issues.

Attitudes to treatment

The Drug Attitude Inventory (DAI) is available in two forms: a 10-item scale and a 30-item scale (Hogan & Awad, 1983). This scale was compiled from service users' statements about antipsychotic medication and has good reliability and validity. The items have a true/false response and are given a +1 or −1 score, depending on whether the response shows a positive or a negative attitude to antipsychotics. The score obtained indicates whether the person has positive or negative attitudes towards their medication. Scores on the DAI have been shown to correlate with biochemical assessments of adherence.

The Attitudes towards Neuroleptic Treatment (ANT) questionnaire (Kampman et al., 2000) consists of 10 attitude statements about neuroleptic treatment and two items for insight on a visual analogue scale. The scale comprises three factors: general attitudes, subjective feeling and expectations, and insight. The authors showed the scale had high inter-item consistency and fair test-retest reliability.

The Rating of Medication Influences (ROMI) scale is a comprehensive scale that assesses attitudinal and behavioural factors influencing adherence with antipsychotic medication (Weiden et al., 1994). It has good psychometric properties, and principal components analysis identified three subscales related to adherence:

- prevention
- influence of others
- medication affinity.

and five subscales relating to non-adherence:

- denial/dysphoria
- logistical problems
- rejection of label
- family influence
- negative therapeutic alliance.

The disadvantage of this scale is that it is lengthy and takes a considerable time to administer. It may be useful to use with particular service users who have problems with adherence in order to identify targets for intervention.

Dolder et al. (2004) developed a shorter eight-item scale, the Brief Evaluation of Medication Influences and Beliefs Scale. This scale showed concurrent validity, correlating with the DAI, adequate internal consistency and significant test-retest reliability for five of the eight items. Its advantages are that it is quick to administer (less than 5 minutes in most cases) and can direct intervention. It is described in more detail in Chapter 6.

The Satisfaction with Information about Medicines Scale (SIMS) was developed by Horne et al. (2001b) to assess service users' satisfaction with information received about their medication. The scale is intended for general use about all medications, but has been used in mental health. The SIMS consists of 17 items split into two subscales:

- action and usage, which includes nine items about how to use medication and what it is prescribed for;
- potential problems of medication, which includes eight items on the adverse effects of medication.

Service users rate the items, indicating their level of satisfaction regarding the information they have been given about their prescribed medication. The scale shows satisfactory internal consistency, test–retest reliability and criterion-related validity. This scale is useful in clinical audit and research, and may be used in clinical practice to identify any dissatisfaction with information provided. Some service users will not indicate voluntarily what information they want to know about medication or they may not expect to be informed about medication, and so this scale can be used to identify areas where more input and explanation are required.

Self-assessment of response to treatment

In addition to the validated measures described above, which can provide a solid basis for prescribing decisions, it is important to focus on the individual service user and how medication is affecting him or her. A reduction in overall KGV scores, for example, may provide comfort to a prescriber but not necessarily the service user.

For example, in the course of a study one service user described how medication had no affect at all on his symptoms. He had experienced negative and abusive auditory hallucinations for many years and after trials of many different antipsychotics and combinations of medication he had never had any relief (Day et al., 1996). However, he stated that he would never stop medication; this seemed to be a paradox. On further questioning, the service user explained that when taking medication he continued to hear voices but that the medication prevented him from being irritable with people around him and getting into arguments. This meant he was better able to continue social contact with people and have a better quality of life despite the medication not having a direct effect on core psychotic symptoms.

It is important to ask people what symptom or side effect most bothers them and to be proactive in targeting those issues that most bother a person. This can have obvious benefits for the service users;

by dealing with the issues that are most pertinent to them, it can have a positive effect on adherence and it can be very rewarding as a health professional.

It can be surprising to find out what bothers individual service users the most, and this is difficult to predict. For example, a service user may be happy to endure what seems a severe or distressing side effect because of the benefits of medication on symptoms. One service user explained that he was not bothered by the 4 stone of weight he had gained since he had been prescribed clozapine because it was the only medication that had ever stopped the voices. Another service user with multiple side effects could tolerate all of the side effects but was extremely distressed by blurred vision, which meant that he could no longer read the *Racing Post*, a pastime he had previously gained great enjoyment from. As part of a randomised controlled trial to improve adherence with medication, a method was developed for people to self-rate symptoms and side effects of medication, which is described in detail elsewhere (Randall et al., 2002). After establishing a rapport and detailed discussion, the service user chooses two or three symptoms and two or three side effects that are most bothersome to them. They can then self-rate these symptoms/side effects every few days and this can chart the impact changes in medication, such as drug choice or dose.

The benefits of self-rating include increased self-efficacy, more awareness of side effects and factors that may impact on symptoms such as stress or exercise, more involvement in treatment and possibly improved attitudes to treatment. For many years in people with disorders such as diabetes, increased self-management of medication has been linked with improvements in health outcomes. Use of self-assessment of symptoms and side effects in mental health could have similar benefits and would fit with current NHS policy.

Conclusion

This chapter has provided an overview of some of the assessment tools that may be useful in evaluating the effects of medication in mental health. In practice, the tools are only an aid to evaluation of the effects of the medication, and open dialogue and listening to the service user's views are the most important part of the process.

When evaluating medication it is important that the service user is fully informed about treatment options and is involved in the choice of medication. Recent policies have all advocated service user involvement in treatment. Research has shown that where service users are fully involved, treatment is better targeted, fewer adverse effects are experienced, and adherence to treatment regimens and treatment outcomes are improved. The treatment prescribed should be effective, and objective assessment of response should be documented. If the treatment is ineffective the treatment should be changed or stopped. This seems obvious and yet in clinical practice some service users are still prescribed high doses of multiple medications with little or no therapeutic benefit and a high burden of adverse effects and increased risk. Whilst evaluation of symptoms is part of the evaluation of a treatment's effects, the effect of medication on overall quality of life is essential. If a treatment completely removes symptoms but the service user is so sedated that he or she is too drowsy to attend college or too embarrassed to go to work because of abnormal movements, then this is not acceptable. We are aiming for recovery, and social functioning is a key aspect of this. The wide range of psychotropic medicines prescribed for mental health problems can cause an array of adverse effects with a negative impact on social functioning, self-esteem and physical health. For example, the atypical antipsychotics that are now widely used, such as clozapine and olanzapine, can cause massive weight gain and this can mean that people avoid social contact, which can exacerbate wellbeing.

Medication in mental health should be tailored to each individual to achieve the most effective treatment possible in terms of reducing symptoms and improving social functioning, and with the fewest adverse effects possible. This will require open dialogue with service users about what they want out of treatment, provision of honest and good quality information about the possible benefits and adverse effects of medication (including that they may not work or only work partially), and a certain amount of trial and error. Assessment tools can facilitate this process but they must be used responsibly and action must be taken on the information they provide.

References

Addington, D., Addington, J. & Maticka-Tyndale, E. (1993) Assessing depression in schizophrenia: The Calgery depression scale. *British Journal of Psychiatry*, **163**(suppl. 22), 39–44.

Andreasen, N.C. (1986) Scale for the assessment of thought, language and communication. *Schizophrenia Bulletin*, **12**(3) 473–482.

American Psychiatric Association (1994) *Diagnostic and Statistical Manual of Mental Disorders*, 4th edn. American Psychiatric Association, Washington, DC.

Andreasen, N.C. (1989) The scale for the Assessment of Negative Symptoms (SANS): Conceptual and theoretical foundations. *British Journal of Psychiatry*, **155**(suppl.), 49–52.

Barnes, T.R. (1989) A rating scale for drug-induced akathisia. *British Journal of Psychiatry*, **154**, 672–676.

Barnes, T.R. (2003) The Barnes Akathisia rating scale – revisited. *Journal of Psychopharmacology*, **17**, 365–370.

Bazaire S. (2007) *Psychotropic Drug Directory*. Healthcomm UK Ltd.

Chaplin, R. & Kent, A. (1998) Informing patients about tardive dyskinesia. *British Journal of Psychiatry*, **172**, 78–81.

Day, J.C., Bentall, R.P. & Warner, S. (1996) Schizophrenic patients' experiences of neuroleptic medication: A Q-methodological investigation. *Acta Psychiatrica Scandinavica*, **93**, 397–402.

Department of Health (2005) *National Health Service Plan*. Department of Health, London.

Department of Health (2006) *Choosing Health: Supporting the physical needs of people with severe mental illness*. Department of Health, London.

Dolder, C.R., Lacro, J.P., Warren, K.A., Golshan, S., Perkins, D.O. & Jeste, D.V. (2004) Brief evaluation of medication influences and beliefs: Development and testing of a brief scale for medication adherence. *Journal of Clinical Psychopharmacology*, **24**, 404–409.

Gabbay, M.B., Shiels, C., Bower, P., Sibbald, B., King, M., & Ward E. (2003) Patient-practitioner agreement: Does it matter? *Psychological Medicine*, **33**, 241–251.

Gruwez, B., Gury, C., Poirier, M.F., et al. (2004) Comparison of two assessment tools of antidepressant side-effects: UKU scale versus spontaneous notification. *Encephale*, **30**(5), 425–432.

Guy, W. (1976) *ECDEU Assessment Manual for Psychopharmacology*, pp. 534–537. US Department of Health Education & Welfare, Washington DC.

Haddock, G., McCarron, J., Tarrier, N. & Faragher, E.B. (1999) Scales to measure dimensions of hallucinations and delusions: The psychotic symptom rating scales (PSYRATS). *Psychological Medicine*, **29**, 879–889.

Haw, C., Stubbs, J., Calton, R. & Haynes, H. (2001) Long-stay psychiatric patients' knowledge and experience in the use of their antipsychotic medication. *Hospital Pharmacist*, **7**, 166–172.

Healthcare Commission State of Health Care (2007) *Improvements and Challenges in Services in England and Wales*. Commission for Healthcare Audit and Inspection, London.

Hogan T.P. & Awad, A.G. (1983) A self-report scale predictive of drug compliance in schizophrenics: reliability and discriminative ability. *Psychological Medicine*, **13**, 177–183.

Horne, R., Frost, S., Hankins, M. & Wright, S. (2001a) 'In the eye of the beholder': pharmacy students have more positive perceptions of medicines than students of other disciplines. *International Journal of Pharmacy Practice*, **9**, 85–89.

Horne, R., Hankins, M. & Jenkins, R. (2001b) The Satisfaction with Information about Medicines Scale (SIMS): A new measurement tool for audit and research. *Quality in Health Care*, **10**, 135–140.

Janno, S., Holi, M.M., Tuisku, K. & Wahbeck, K. (2005) Validity of the Simpson-Angus Scale (SAS) in a naturalistic schizophrenia population. *BMC Neurology*, **5**, 5.

Jones, P.B., Barnes, T.R.E., Davies, L., et al. (2006) Randomized controlled trial of the effect on quality of life of second vs. first generation antipsychotic drugs in schizophrenia. *Archives of General Psychiatry*, **63**, 1079–1087.

Jung, H.Y., Kim, J.H., Ahn, Y.M., Kim, S.C., Hwang, S.S. & Kim, Y.S. (2005) Liverpool University Neuroleptic Side Effect Rating Scale (LUNSERS) as a subjective measure of drug-induced Parkinsonism and akathisia. *Human Psychopharmacology*, **20**, 41–45.

Junghan, U.M., Leese, M., Priebe, S., & Slade, M. (2007) Staff and patient perspectives on unmet need and therapeutic alliance in community mental health services. *British Journal of Psychiatry*, **191**, 543–547.

Kampman, O., Lehtinen, K., Lassila, V., Leinonen, E., Poutanen, O. & Koivisto, A. (2000) Attitudes towards neuroleptic treatment: Reliability and validity of the Attitudes towards Neuroleptic Treatment (ANT) questionnaire. *Schizophrenia Research*, **45**, 223–234.

Kraweika, M., Goldberg, D.P. & Vaughn, M. (1977) A standardized psychiatric assessment scale for rating Chronic Psychiatric Patients. *Acta Psychiatrica Scandinavica*, **55**, 299–308.

Lader, M. (1999) Some adverse effects of antipsychotics: prevention and treatment. *Journal of Clinical Psychiatry*, **60**(Suppl 12), 18–21.

Lasalvia, A., Bonetto, C., Tansella, M., Stefani, B., & Ruggeri, M. (2008) Does staff–patient agreement on needs for care predict a better mental health outcome? A 4-year follow-up in a community service. *Psychological Medicine*, **38**, 123–33.

Lingjaerde, O., Ahlfors, U.G., Bech, P., Dencker, S.J., & Elgen, K. (1987) The UKU side effect rating scale. A new comprehensive rating scale for psychotropic drugs and a cross-sectional study of side effects in neuroleptic-treated patients. *Acta Psychiatrica Scandinavica,* **334**, 1–100.

Mackell, J.A., Harrison, D.J. & McDonnell, D.D. (2005) Relationship between preventative physical health care and mental health in individuals with schizophrenia: a survey of caregivers *Mental Health Services Research,* **7**(4), 225–228.

Macpherson, R., Jerrom, B. & Hughes, A. (1996) A controlled study of education about drug treatment in schizophrenia. *British Journal of Psychiatry*, **168**, 709–717.

Mitchell, A.J. & Malone, D. (2006) Physical health and schizophrenia. *Current Opinion in Psychiatry*, **19**, 432–437.

Munetz, M.R. & Benjamin, S. (1988) How to examine patients using the abnormal involuntary movement scale. *Hospital and Community Psychiatry*, **39**, 1172–1177.

National Institute of Clinical Excellence (2002) *Schizophrenia, Core Interventions in the Treatment and Management of Schizophrenia in Primary and Secondary Care*. Department of Health, London.

Osborn, D.P.J., King, M.B. & Nazareth, I. (2003) Participation in screening for cardiovascular risk by people with schizophrenia or similar mental illnesses: Cross sectional study in general practice. *British Medical Journal,* **326**, 1122–1123.

Penedoa, F.R. & Dahn, J.R. (2005) Exercise and well-being: A review of mental and physical health benefits associated with physical activity. *Current Opinion in Psychiatry,* **18**, 189–193.

Phelan, M., Stradins, L. & Morrison, S. (2001) Physical health of people with severe mental illness. *British Medical Journal,* **322**, 443–444.

Randall, F., Wood, P., Day, J. Bentall, R.P., Rogers, A. & Healy, D. (2002) Enhancing appropriate adherence with neuroleptic medication: two contrasting approaches. In: Morrison, T. (ed.) *A Case Book of Cognitive Therapy for Psychosis*. Psychology Press, Brighton.

Rege, S. (2008) Antipsychotic induced weight gain in schizophrenia: Mechanisms and management. *Australian and New Zealand Journal of Psychiatry,* **42**, 369–381.

Roberts, L., Roalfe, A., Wilson, S. & Lester, H. (2007) Physical health care of patients with schizophrenia in primary care: a comparative study. *Family Practice,* **24**, 34–40.

Sachdev, P.S. (1994) A rating scale for acute drug-induced akathisia: development, reliability and validity. *Biological Psychiatry,* **35**, 263–271.

Simpson, G. & Angus, J. (1970) A rating scale for extrapyramidal side effects. *Acta Psychiatrica Scandinavica,* **44**, 11–19.

Waddington, J.L., Youssef, H.A. & Kinsella, A. (1998) Mortality in schizophrenia antipsychotic polypharmacy and absence of adjunctive anticholinergics over the course of a 10 year prospective study. *British Journal of Psychiatry,* **173**, 325–329.

Wadell, L. & Taylor, M. (2008) A new self-rating scale for detecting atypical or second-generation antipsychotic side effects. *Journal of Psychopharmacology,* **22**(3), 238–243.

Weiden, P., Rapkin, B., Mott, T., et al. (1994) Rating of medication influences (ROMI) scale in schizophrenia. *Schizophrenia Bulletin,* **20**, 297–310.

Young R.C., Biggs J.T., Ziegler V.E. & Meyer D.A. (1978) A rating scale for mania: reliability, validity and sensitivity. *British Journal of Psychiatry,* **133**, 429–435.

Yusufi, B.Z., Mukherjee, S., Aitchison, K., Dunn, G., Page, E., & Barnes, T.R.E. (2005) Reliability of the antipsychotic non-neurological side-effects rating scale (ANNSERS). *Journal of Psychopharmacology,* **19**(Suppl.), A10.

Zigmond, A.S. & Snaith, R.P. (1983) The hospital anxiety and depression scale. *Acta Psychiatrica Scandinavica,* **67**, 361–370.

Exploring medication issues with service users – achieving concordance

Neil Harris

Introduction

Enabling people to be prescribed their optimum medication regimen, with the provision of arrangements for administration, and help them become self-efficacious in the management of pharmacological treatment are the goals of medicines management work. These aims benefit both those whose medication regimen is working well and people who have problems with pharmacological treatment.

In this chapter, a range of interventions and strategies are described that help people to explore their medication experiences and develop understanding, which:

- enables the person to make an informed decision about medication;
- enables them to engage in shared decision-making about medication;
- provides information that enables the person to receive the medication that suits him or her best – given the subjective nature of the effects of psychotropic medication.

One of the values of a comprehensive and individualised medicines management programme is that it can provide increased skills and knowledge that enable people to use medication as part of their recovery. The positive, personal outcomes of successful medicines management can include increased self-efficacy by mastery of symptoms and relapse prevention, as well as a psychological boost in terms of developing confidence and self-esteem by demonstrating abilities in practical and negotiation skills.

Nevertheless, people will develop their own priority for this kind of work, other agendas, difficulties and needs, both long-term and

189

immediate. Also, the value people place on discussion about medication will be based on how useful the drugs are and the perceived response from the care team and family members. Practitioners need to be flexible, and sometimes it is more useful to take a longer view about engaging service users in medicines management than completing a comprehensive programme.

This chapter provides a range of interventions that can help people to explore the effects of medication, treatment issues and their experience of services, create long- and short-term treatment goals, and overcome difficulties. To this end it provides a framework for developing meaningful work with service users: a focused therapeutic dialogue. The chapter aims to provide information which represents good practice, and directs the reader to employ ways of working which helps people to work collaboratively in making informed decisions about what medicines they are prepared to take. This 'shared decision-making' or concordance is an alliance, a partnership, where an agreement is made regarding how medication will be used to address difficulties and aid recovery.

Throughout this chapter, reference is made to working with service users but, wherever possible and appropriate, work in this area should include relatives and carers. Involving significant others in the medication management of their relative or friend is an essential element in enabling effective care by harnessing their unique expertise and knowledge. Involvement in this process enables relatives and carers to gain fuller understanding and information regarding the person's mental health condition, contribute to planning, intervention and evaluation, and voice their needs for information and support (National Institute for Mental Health in England, 2005).

Strategies for helping service users develop an understanding about the role of medication and how it can help them

The process of work in medication management is tailored to the service user. Plans are based on standardised and informal assessment information, prescription history, personal accounts and expressed needs of service users, carers and other sources of information, together with theoretical and research information about medicines, their actions, uses and complications. The resulting individualised profile is an amalgam of medication effects (positive and negative), personal beliefs and the influences of others. It forms the basis for discussions and decisions about prioritising work, setting goals and developing care plans, and it guides decisions about the methods and interventions most likely to result in the achievement of goals.

By developing understanding and knowledge about their psycho-tropic medication and treatment influences, people will be increasingly informed to take an active part in treatment decisions but may find it difficult to talk about their treatment to members of the care team. It will be useful, therefore, to look at how the person's abilities can be enhanced in this area before describing the strategies more closely.

Developing the skills to become effective negotiators of health care

Developing the confidence and skills to take an active part in treatment decisions may take some time to achieve, given the hierarchical nature of relationships between mental health practitioners and the service users and their carers. Past experiences, where practitioners may have taken a lead role in consultation, and cultural expectations to follow their instructions may have had a negative effect on people's perception of not only their role in the process, but their rights to be involved.

Collaborative working is about openly and honestly sharing infor-mation, and ensuring full discussions on aspects that are important to the service user. People should feel they are active partners in treatment decisions and have influence regarding the frequency and format of treatment reviews.

There are some useful steps that can be taken to help the person become effective in meetings with prescribers:

* identify the person's objectives for the next consultation and plan how these are going to be communicated in the meeting;
* rehearse and role-play the points the person wants to get across;
* write things down; record the things the person wants to say and take notes about what is said;
* list the questions the person wants to ask. Useful questions include:
  * Is the dose of medication safe for me?
  * How long will I have to take medication – when will I be able to come off the medicine?
  * How will the medication affect me, physically and psychologically?
  * How much alcohol can I drink whilst on the medication?
  * What are the effects if I find out I am pregnant?
  * Can I become dependent on the medication?
  * How does it affect other medicines I am taking?
  * Are there alternative treatments if I decide that I don't want to take this kind of medication?

(Department of Health, 2008)

It is important to provide the person with support and advocacy. Talk about the meeting afterwards, the things that went well or not so well, how the person felt. Providing feedback can be useful, and identifying and commending effective strategies and interactions should form part of this.

Giving information

People's beliefs about medication are the single most important factor in their decision about whether or not to take medication and, if they do decide to take it, when and how. Yet the perspectives that validate people's decisions will be a combination of many personal factors: experience of symptoms and their consequences, subjective experience of the medication, perceived risks, experience of services, carers' views, culture, knowledge, current circumstances, anxiety, fear and distress. The decisions people come to may be based on a mistaken or incomplete understanding of mental illness or the use and utility of medication or based on their experience of what medicines are useful, in what dose, at what time, in what circumstances.

Service users and carers have been asking for clear, unbiased information about medicines for some time. There can be an expectation that the service user needs to be proactive in finding useful information rather than practitioners viewing information giving as an important part of their role. Frequently the information sheet that comes with the medicine is inadequate or unclear and prompts questions rather than answers them. Furthermore, unpleasant experiences can be attributed to a person's illness rather than the side effects of medication, misdirecting decision-making.

The collaborative nature of working with people indicates that they should be fully informed about the likely effects of their medication, and be encouraged to ask questions about their medication and alternative treatments. For example, a study by Chaplin & Kent (1998) suggested that, although it was safe to inform services users about tardive dyskinesia (TD), there is the possibility of generating alarm and anger when informing people who have been receiving these drugs for a lengthy period.

Exercises to aid understanding and decision-making

Looking back – doing a timeline

This exercise can be useful in helping people to engage in medication-centred work. It involves recollecting life experiences whilst maintaining a focus on treatment, effects of medication, involvement with services, significant events and people. Looking for events and patterns, antecedents and consequences, stress points and good times, effective and ineffective strategies are all things that can help people identify their personal factors which have an effect on staying well or becoming unwell.

Starting from the onset of mental health problems, detail can be given through discussions with the service user and significant others, and more detail added in the time between meetings. The construction of this biography can continue over time and the person can gain useful insights regarding the effect of individual medications, the consequences of adherence and discontinuation and the link between stressful life events and becoming unwell. Adding further value to this work would be a detailed prescription history, which should inform future changes to medication regimens by providing clear information about what has been tried in the past and the reasons for discontinuation.

Checking the pros and cons of medication

Most people have a range of ideas, experiences and beliefs which play a role in their decision regarding whether they should take or not take medication. This exercise aims to focus on these by exploring what are the good and bad things about taking or discontinuing medication. The balance between the advantages and disadvantages of taking medication can be a fine one. Side effects can be as disturbing as the symptoms they treat. By exploring the reasons that have guided people's decisions about medicines, it maybe shown that their standpoint is not based on a single belief or idea but is often made up from a number of positive and negative ideas. People may feel uncertain or ambivalent about taking medication, and actively exploring these ideas is not only useful in helping the person to develop an informed decision about taking or not taking the medication, but can often identify inconsistencies that can be gently explored and lead to reappraisal of medication taking.

Looking forward

Goal setting is an important aspect of everyday life, and making it enables plans to be made for the future. In recognising the part that medication plays in achieving the goals, it is important to emphasise the long-term role medication may play in helping the person get to where he or she wants to be. Whether it is staying well, finding a new job or accommodation, or taking a holiday, questions can be asked: What things need to happen in order for these goals to be achieved? What has been helpful in the past? How can medication help to achieve this goal? When the goal has been clearly defined, problem-solving can be used to identify the steps which will be needed (due to the importance of this intervention it has been given its own chapter). Planning for the future has beneficial effects in terms of improving the person's confidence in his or her ability to make changes for the better, drawing attention to actions which result in positive change, and it reframes medication as an aid to goal achievement rather than hindrance.

Working with beliefs about medication

Over time, through getting to know the person and engaging in information-giving sessions, the views and beliefs he or she has about medication may be presented for discussion. Beliefs are based on a complex mixture of a person's characteristics and his or her experience. They can include factors such as:

- the subjective effects of medication;
- the person's belief about self-sufficiency and self-reliance;
- contact with services and individual practitioners;
- the advice of close friends and family;
- the person's perception about the mental health problems they have;
- the person's cultural perspective on taking medication.

Like all beliefs they may be resistant to change and the person will be biased towards evidence that confirms the 'truth' of their belief. It is known that the certainty a person has about a belief can vary; conviction can vary over time and not all beliefs are held with 100% certainty.

Work in this area is difficult and requires sensitivity; very strongly held beliefs are unlikely to be affected by intervention and the therapeutic relationship could suffer if the person feels threatened by pressure. However, if it is felt that useful work can be undertaken then this four-stage model is useful (Everitt & Siddle, 2002):

- Take time to describe the belief clearly and completely, ensuring collaborative agreement.
- Ask the person to rate the level of conviction with which the belief is held (from 0% not true to 100% completely convinced).
- Collect and explore the evidence on which the belief is based.
- Re-rate the conviction.

Some useful good practice points include:

- It is not useful to challenge the belief itself.
- Beliefs are a way of trying to make sense of what is happening – reasonable and understandable.

- Beliefs may be linked to distress and disturbance.
- Listen for themes and inconsistencies.
- If people want to convince the practitioner of the veracity of their beliefs it is sometimes useful to agree to differ or suspend disbelief (Kingdon & Turkington, 1994).

Advanced directives

As part of this work it may be useful to develop 'advanced directives', sometimes called a 'living will' (Care Services Improvement Partnership, 2002). This is a document made when the person is well and states what treatment and care the person wants should he or she become ill and lack the capacity to make informed treatment decisions. The directive can indicate medication that has helped in the past and highlight drugs to avoid. It can include information about who to contact and what to tell them and who the person wants to act on their behalf. Work in this area is useful, not only from a practical perspective of providing useful information regarding prescribing for the person in an emergency, but in emphasising a person's need and right to become involved in treatment decisions. Construction of an advanced directive has been positively valued by service users (Sutherby et al., 1999) and demonstrates a tangible example of their involvement. It also requires the person to reflect on and evaluate his or her care and treatment, both necessary features of concordance.

The structure and components of a medication management session

Good practice points in developing useful discussions about medication

Before looking at a framework to plan and deliver a medication management session it will be useful to briefly mention some key pointers in engaging people in discussions about their medication and to develop motivation to become proactive, skilful and effective in their treatment management.

There are some features about sessions with service users that can maximise the effectiveness of medication management and others which impede progress.

Provide positive statements for undertaking medication management work

It is important to use and create opportunities to commend people for expressing their attitudes, beliefs and ideas, and demonstrating practical actions in medication management. Examples of communications and acts that should attract positive comments would include a willingness to discuss sensitive or difficult issues, additions to timelines and pros and cons of work, suggestions and requests for future work, work accomplished between meetings, developments in the person's self-efficacy, and generally any behaviours which indicate a proactive stance towards medication management work. This emphasis will develop people's self-confidence in managing their medication, highlight their contribution to positive outcomes and demonstrate the autonomy they have in their care. In this sense it is important to identify the things that have been useful and worked well, things that are in the person's control and influence, avoiding discussions about 'failure' and what the person 'did wrong'.

Have a conversation

When practitioners first use the medication management checklist (Appendix 11.1), it can feel as though their interactions have become wooden, unnatural, as if the checklist imposes a session format that is too formal and cold. Over time, experience of working in this way enables the practitioner to conduct an organised, well-planned session, adopting an interactive style that reflects their way of being with a person. Good practices and appropriate interventions can be incorporated which focus sessions in a useful way for the service user.

Work with clear aims, collaboratively created

Developing clear and collaborative long- and short-term aims is important in planning work and ensuring that there is a common understanding about not only the direction and content of work but importantly the benefit and value of the work. This work will link sessions together, emphasising the continuity of work in this area and will be enhanced with the use of summaries and reviews of previous work.

Work to the person's timescale

It is important to remember that the person will have different priorities and competing claims for time, and the practitioners wish to 'get through' a medication management programme may not be shared by the service user. Pacing the work to suit what the person wants and needs develops the collaborative ethos that is required to achieve concordance. As Repper and Perkins (2003) put it, practitioners need to be 'on-tap, not on top'. It is also important to remember that for long-term mental health problems practitioners and service users need to take a long-term perspective; change sometime occurs slowly and imperceptibly and this can easily lead to demoralisation and reduced motivation. Short-term goal planning offers an incremental approach to progress and development and enables people to perceive their lives as changing rather than static. This can be reflected and reinforced by visible changes in assessment and timeline data.

Developing connections

In discussing the effects of medication it is important to review the person's treatment history to explore the connections between taking, or not taking, medication, prescription changes and changes in personal circumstances. Is there a link between taking medication and relapse? How did the person feel as a result of his or her decision to discontinue? Is the dose too much or too little? How does the person's relationships change as a result of taking medication? Has medication helped in getting through stressful periods? The answers to these and other questions help the person to develop a body of evidence on which to base future decisions.

The Medication Management Checklist (Harris, 2008)

Planning and structuring session time with service users goes some way to making the most efficient use of time working on medication management. The checklist provided can be used to develop the structure and content of sessions with service users. This checklist has been modified from a validated scale developed by Haddock et al. (2001) for assessing the skills of cognitive behaviour therapy (CBT) therapists and is divided into two parts: general skills and specialist medication management components. The general skills are those areas of practice considered to be common components of good therapeutic work and this part retains the sections and items found in the original scale. In the specialist medication management part there are three sections which aim to encompass the range of work involved in medication management: evaluating experience, the person's ability to take medication and consent. The specialist part has also retained the sections on guided discovery and work between meetings as they form an integral part of medicines management.

The specialist section was initially developed using material from good practice guidelines, academic papers and expert opinion. As a result of using the checklist to assess and supervise students undertaking an undergraduate medicines management module, and taking into account discussions with course staff and a multidisciplinary group of supervisors, the checklist has undergone a number of revisions. These changes sought to identify and remove ambiguities and inconstancies whilst developing clarity and accuracy, ensuring completeness of the process of medication management and improving the ease of use.

In the version presented in Appendix 11.1, both general and specialist medication management sections correspond to the themes and items found in the *Competency Framework for Shared Decision-Making with Patients* developed by the National Prescribing Centre (2007). Taking all these factors together, the checklist can be said to have good face validity. Anecdotal evidence indicates that the checklist may have good inter-rater reliability, although this has not been formally tested.

The checklist can be used in a number of ways across a wide range of clinical situations and with a variety of service user groups:

Develop practice	Helping the practitioner to develop an effective format for delivering a medication management session
Supervision	To be used as a focus for supervision sessions, ideally with an audio recording of a session with a person
Skills assessment	As part of a training programme, using role play and rehearsed practice
Planning work	To develop the content of a session, focusing on the different aspects of medication management

Part 1: General skills

Agenda setting

After checking that the person is emotionally able to attend to the focus of the meeting, the setting of an agenda should be undertaken early in the session. This is a collaborative process and should not be simply a procedure for practitioners to seek approval for their agenda items. It should reflect a realistic amount of work for the time allotment and needs to include any relevant events that the person has experienced since the last meeting.

Feedback

Feedback, both positive and negative, regarding previous and current sessions needs to be sought: Was the work helpful? Any areas which could improve the effectiveness of the work? Is the person clear about the purpose of the work and its implications? Answers to these questions can help to fine-tune sessions and summaries, and can clarify understanding of the practitioner's role and expectations.

Understanding

Developing and conveying understanding uses summaries and re-phrasing of discussions. Sensitivity and empathy are required to be effective in this area and it is important to be mindful of comments that might negate the person's views. Differences in viewpoint will occur. Acknowledgement and respect for these divergent views and recognition of the person's view is an important part of the therapeutic process.

Interpersonal effectiveness

Interpersonal effectiveness can be shown by being open, honest and caring, answering questions and, where appropriate, using humour. Comments voicing criticism or disapproval are counter-productive to the therapeutic relationship and can be interpreted as invalidating work undertaken. Another aspect of proficiency in this area is to enable a dialogue that results in a balance between listening and talking, where the discussion is not dominated by the practitioner or service user, but an inter-change of information can be achieved.

Collaboration

Collaboration is the cornerstone of effective work towards concordance, self-efficacy in illness management and recovery. Opportunities should be used to cement the person's involvement in medicines management, offering choices, asking for and acknowledging suggestions and ways forward. A key feature of the work is the presentation of a rationale: a clear and practical reason for undertaking the work or task which the person can see fits in with the goals of medicines management and provides a logical link to the agreed goals. The rationale should also include an explanation for the use of particular interventions and strategies.

Finally, successful work in medication management is dependent on the practitioner's use of clear, jargon-free language, and an awareness of the use of technical terminology and abbreviations is needed to ensure the person can engage in work.

Part 2: Specific medication management items

At the beginning of this part of the checklist, a statement acknowledges that work in these areas can take some time to complete and that individual sessions will be targeted on certain aspects of management. Whereas all work will require the use of the general skills, as well as 'guided discovery' and 'agreeing work between sessions' in the specialist part, the content or agenda for a session will focus on one of the specific areas of management.

Evaluating the service user's experience of medication

This section explores the effectiveness of medication in symptom control, side-effect experience and arrangements for monitoring. It looks at lifestyle issues and how they inter-relate with medication. Questions are asked about the circumstances around previous medication changes and the need for potential changes in the future.

Assessing and enhancing the person's ability to take medication

Here, work seeks to identify the difficulties and positives strategies the person has regarding taking medication. It focuses not only on the practical aspects of obtaining and taking medicines but the resources, supports and assets the person has. Difficulties are addressed with reference to problem solving. In this section, personal beliefs about medication are explored; this is a key factor in adherence and concordance.

Addressing consent

The checklist takes account of the varying needs that people have regarding information about treatment and diagnosis, by enquiring about the person's current levels of knowledge, perceived gaps in knowledge and the provision of information. It addresses the other components of valid consent, the absence of coercion, the issue of capacity and asks whether the person has agreed to take the prescribed medicines. Questions are asked to determine whether the person has any difficulties in expressing his or her needs or taking part in shared decision-making. Finally, feedback is sought regarding strategies for change and support.

The two sections retained from the original scale are now described.

Guided discovery

A useful way of thinking about guided discovery is to liken it to an investigatory communication style (like that of TV cop Columbo). Questions are used to help the service users 'discover' and explore their ideas and beliefs about treatment and treatment experiences, as opposed to the practitioner trying to persuading them to adopt a point of view. The practitioner encourages the service users to explore or question aspects of their treatment needs or to review past experiences or to make connections between treatment and distressing illness experiences.

Guided discovery uses a lot of techniques and methods in order to facilitate this investigatory process, including behavioural experiments, between session tasks, clarification and use of summaries, and Socratic dialogue.

Socratic dialogue is a questioning style where the practitioner uses a series of open-ended questions to lead the service users to examine incongruities and inconsistencies, or arbitrary conclusions and assumptions regarding their attitudes and opinions regarding medication. Questions are used to:

- clarify meaning;
- identify thoughts, ideas, assumption and beliefs;
- examine the effects of medication;
- examine the meaning of events;
- explore relationships;
- examine the consequences of certain actions and decisions.

Socratic dialogue attempts to promote curiosity in people, encouraging them to stand back and re-evaluate their experiences in an objective manner, examining both sides of an argument.

The technique uses general questions (when? what? how? why? who?) followed by more probing questions to elicit detail, taking care to only include questions that the person can answer. The questions should open up subject areas, not close them down. Work can progress from attention, to concrete aspects of medication and treatment, to more abstract issues. The process can enable the person to generalise this new method of personal evaluation to other areas of his or her life. This can result in the re-evaluation of previous conclusions and the development of new ways of thinking to improve future problem solving and concept formation.

The effectiveness of this way of working depends on the communication skills and style of the practitioner, who must be genuinely seeking to understand the person's views and experiences. People should not feel as though they are being interrogated, and the development of good listening and summarising skills are essential components of guided discovery (Padesky, 1993; Fowler et al., 1995).

Agreeing work between sessions

Undertaking work between meetings (homework) is an integral part of medication management and aims to enable the person to gather new information and test new skills and ideas. Between session tasks are generated collaboratively, building on rationales identified in working together and geared towards enabling service users to make progress in developing self-efficacy and increase understanding of their mental health problem and treatment. Between session tasks are important in maintaining the learning process. Work can include:

- completing a questionnaire, like the LUNSERS;
- monitoring symptoms to measure the efficacy of medication;
- reading an information leaflet or website or watching a DVD;

- using a new administration regimen to check its effectiveness;
- adding detail to a history or beliefs exercise, like the timeline or pros and cons;
- exploring the evidence for the efficacy of medication;
- generating a list of solutions to a particular problem.

The balance of work is important, and to get this right can be difficult. Too much or too difficult work can become a burden or overwhelming, too little may be perceived as a waste of time or meaningless, leaving the person with a sense of failure or letting down the practitioner. Once agreed it is useful to write the task down for the service users to take with them and should conform to the SMART formula (specific, measurable, achievable, relevant and time limited). Obstacles to completing the task can be identified and solutions found in a collaborative manner.

It is important that the work is keyed into the aims and goals of the session and the person's efforts should be reviewed and discussed early in the next session, maximising the gains made, reinforcing his or her efforts and demonstrating progress toward self-efficacy.

It must not be forgotten that undertaking tasks between sessions is not the sole preserve of the service user and it may well be the case that decisions involve the practitioner taking responsibility for actively completing tasks before the next session.

Finally, an opportunity is provided to make a judgement about the overall quality of the medication management session. This assessment is made using a six-point scale from 'barely adequate' to 'excellent'.

Conclusion

In this chapter we have looked at some of the ways service users can explore the experience of pharmaceutical treatment, the effects of their medicines and how they can be used in recovery, involving services, and the influence of family and friends. A checklist has been described, providing a structure to guide the format and content of medicines management sessions. Given that individuals often have competing demands on time, the checklist can help to make the most efficient use of medicines management work.

Working with people and their families to derive maximum benefit from medicines takes skill and knowledge. Many medication management education programmes have been developed, incorporating supervision, and practitioners would be advised to access training in this area.

Appendix 11.1 Medication management session checklist

Coding key:

0 = inappropriately omitted
1 = appropriately included
9 = not applicable (carries a score of 1)

I GENERAL
a) Agenda
   1 The practitioner noted person's current emotional status regarding agenda setting.
   2 Practitioner and service user established agenda for session.
   3 Priorities for agenda items were established.
   4 Agenda was appropriate for time allotment (neither too ambitious nor too limited).
   5 The agenda provided an opportunity for the person to discuss salient events or problems occurring during the time since the last session.
   6 The agenda was adhered to during the session where appropriate.
b) Feedback
   1 The practitioner asked for feedback regarding previous session.
   2 Practitioner asked for feedback and reactions to present session.
   3 Practitioner asked the service user specifically for any *negative* reactions to the practitioner, content, formulation, etc.
   4 Practitioner attempted to respond to the person's feedback.
   5 Practitioner checked that the service user clearly understood the practitioner's role and/or the purpose and limitations of sessions.
   6 Practitioner checked that s/he had fully understood the person's perspective by summarising and asking person to fine-tune or correct as appropriate.
c) Understanding
   1 Practitioner conveys understanding by rephrasing or summarising what the person had said.
   2 Practitioner shows sensitivity, e.g. by reflecting back feelings as well as ideas.
   3 Practitioner's tone of voice was empathic.
   4 Practitioner acknowledged person's viewpoint as valid and important.
   5 Practitioner did not negate person's point of view.
   6 Where differences occurred, they were acknowledged and respected.

Continued

d) Interpersonal effectiveness
1 Practitioner seemed open rather than defensive, shown by not holding back impressions or information nor evading service user's questions.
2 Content of what practitioner said communicated warmth, concern and caring, rather than cold indifference.
3 The practitioner did not criticise, disapprove or ridicule the person's behaviour or point of view.
4 The practitioner responded to, or displayed, humour when appropriate.
5 Practitioner made clear statements without frequent hesitations or rephrasing.
6 Practitioner was in control of the session; s/he was able to shift appropriately between listening and leading.

e) Collaboration
1 Practitioner asked the service user for suggestions on how to proceed and offered choices when feasible.
2 Practitioner ensured that person's suggestions and choices were acknowledged.
3 Practitioner explained rationale for intervention(s).
4 Flow of verbal interchange was smooth, with a balance of listening and talking.
5 Practitioner worked with the person even when using a primarily educative role.
6 Discussion was pitched at a level and in a language that was understandable by the service user.

II Specific medication management items

A medication management package can take a number of sessions to deliver. This part of the scale focuses on the process issues of medication management.

In conducting a medication management focused session *practitioners* should be cognisant to the weight of time given to individual sections within this checklist.

Not all areas of work within the specific medication management section of the checklist should be included within an individual medication management session. For example, the planned session may be evaluating symptom control or side-effect assessment and this would form the main content of a session, therefore the 'Evaluating current medication regimen' (g) section in the checklist, together with the general section, would be used to evaluate that particular session.

However, 'agreeing work between sessions' and items within 'guided discovery' should be included in every session.

Continued

f) Guided discovery
   1 The practitioner used questions to elicit key influences in making medication-related decisions.
   2 The practitioner used questions to determine the beliefs and/or concerns a person, or others involved in their care, has toward medication.
   3 The practitioner used questions to develop the person's understanding of their medication-related behaviour and/or attitudes they have towards medication.
   4 The practitioner used questions to help the person explore problem(s) and/or benefits of medication and management.
   5 The practitioner used questions to consider alternative perspectives regarding medication.
   6 The practitioner used questions to elicit ways of solving a problem and/or planning for the future.
g) Evaluating the service user's experience of medication
   1 Questioning or intervention(s) were used to determine the effectiveness of medication in symptom management.
   2 Used questioning to establish the presence and extent of side effects and/or agreement was reached regarding assessment of side effects.
   3 Used questions to ascertain the person's circumstances or lifestyle choices that may affect the medication.
   4 Discussed ideas regarding treatment changes which may be/or have been required **and/or** side-effect management.
   5 A discussion took place regarding strategies and interventions for management.
   6 Discussions took place regarding the monitoring of persistent symptoms and/or effects of medication.
h) Assessing and enhancing the person's ability to take medication
   1 Practitioner's questions to identify details regarding difficulties and/or positive strategies employed in taking medication.
   2 A problem-solving process is collaboratively undertaken.
   3 The person's beliefs about medication were explored.
   4 The current method of obtaining the person's medication was discussed.
   5 The current method of administering the person's medication was discussed.
   6 The practitioner asked questions to establish the range and extent of help and support the service user has.
i) Addressing consent
   1. The practitioner:
      a) asks questions to ascertain the person's knowledge about their medication and/or diagnosis or;

Continued

b)   enquires whether the person needs any information about their medication **and/or** diagnosis or;

c)   provides information about their medication **and/or** diagnosis in an appropriate way.

2.   The practitioner enquires whether the person agrees to take the prescribed medication.

3.   Practitioner enquires whether the person feels pressured into taking medication.

4.   The practitioner asks questions to ascertain the person's ability to:

a.   understand the nature and purpose of the recommended treatment;

b.   weigh the consequences of having or not having the recommended treatment;

c.   use the medication-related information to form a reasoned judgement regarding treatment.

5.   The practitioner asks questions to ascertain problems the person may have in expressing their preferences and difficulties regarding their treatment.

6.   Practitioner sought adequate feedback from the person regarding the strategy for change and/or support.

j)   Agreeing work between sessions

1   Practitioner explicitly reviewed previous medication-related work.

2   A discussion took place to summarise conclusions derived, or progress made, from this work.

3   Understanding regarding the benefit of the tasks was established.

4   The person and/or practitioner agreed their respective tasks.

5   Goals were defined with the SMART framework: specific, measurable, attainable, realistic and time-framed.

6   A discussion took place to anticipate any problems that may occur in carrying out the tasks, including the need for written details if appropriate.

k)   Quality of medication management interactions

The session was conducted at a level that was:

1   barely adequate

2   mediocre

3   satisfactory

4   good

5   very good

6   excellent

(Reproduced with permission of Gillian Haddock (Haddock et al., 2001)

References

Care Services Improvement Partnership (2002) *Advance Directives, Statements and Agreements and Crisis Cards.* www.schizophreniaguidelines.co.uk/ users_carers/advance_directives.php.

Chaplin, R. & Kent, A. (1998) Informing patients about tardive dyskinesia. *British Journal of Psychiatry,* **172**, 78–81.

Department of Health (2008) *Medicines Management: Everybody's Business. A guide for Service Users, Carers and Health and Social Care Practitioners.* Department of Health, London.

Everitt, J. & Siddle, R. (2002) *Assessment and Therapeutic Interventions with Positive Psychotic Symptoms*, p. 108. In: Harris, N., Williams, S. & Bradshaw, T.) *Psychological Interventions for People with Schizophrenia.* Palgrave, Basingstoke.

Fowler, D., Garety, P. & Kuipers, E. (1995) *Cognitive Behaviour Therapy for Psychosis*, p. 129. Wiley, Chichester.

Haddock, G., Devane, S., Bradshaw, T., et al. (2001) An investigation into the psychometric properties of the cognitive therapy scale for psychosis (CTS-Psy) *Behavioural and Cognitive Psychotherapy,* **29**, 221–233.

Harris, N. (2008) *Medication Management Session Checklist.* University of Manchester, Manchester.

Kingdon, D. & Turkington, D. (1994) *Cognitive Behavioural Therapy for Schizophrenia*, p. 149. Pub. The Guilford Press, Hove.

National Institute for Mental Health in England (2005) *Valuing Carers.* National Institute for Mental Health in England, London.

National Prescribing Centre (2007) *A Competency Framework for Shared Decision-making with Patients; Achieving Concordance for Taking Medicines.* National Prescribing Centre, London.

Padesky, C.A. (1993) *Keynote Address – European Congress of Behavioural and Cognitive Therapies*, London.

Repper, J. & Perkins, R. (2003) *Social Inclusion and Recovery.* Balliere Tindall, London.

Sutherby, K., Szmukler, G., Halpern, A., Alexander, M., Thornicroft, G., & Johnson, C. (1999) A study of 'crisis cards' in a community psychiatric service. *Acta Psychiatrica Scandinavica,* **100**, 56–61.

Problem solving in medicines management

John Baker and Janine Fletcher

Introduction

This chapter begins by providing an overview of some of the common problems and issues that arise with medication. The chapter reviews the history of problem solving as a clinical intervention and then highlights some of the current evidence base before detailing the process of problem solving. The authors then propose that the technique of problem solving is a commonly used, evidence-based, brief intervention, and can be effective in the management of medication issues. The chapter concludes with a fictitious case study, which explores the application of problem solving in a primary care clinical scenario relating to medication management.

Common problems associated with medication

There is a robust evidence base for the role of medication for a variety of mental health problems. However, it is also well documented that many patients do not take their medication as directed. In fact, since 1975 more than 200 reasons for patients not taking medication have been proposed (Vermeire et al., 2001). The issues associated with non-adherence have been categorised into three main categories: side effects, concerns about medication and practical aspects (Barber et al., 2004). Barber and colleagues found that these issues resulted in a third of patients not continuing with their treatment, either intentionally or unintentionally, by day 10 of treatment. In addition, health professionals' attitudes and lack of information can cause additional problems to service user experiences of prescribed medication.

Table 12.1 An overview of common problems associated with medication

Type of problem	Examples
i. Issues associated with health professionals	Review of medication regimes Access to GP or psychiatrist Inconsistencies of staff
ii. Practical issues associated with obtaining medication	Getting repeat prescriptions Getting to the pharmacy Cost, paying for prescriptions
iii. Practical issues associated with taking medication	Remembering to take medication Swallowing tablets Halving them if necessary
iv. Effects and side effects of medication	*'They make me drowsy'* *'I put weight on'*
v. Knowledge and information needs	What the medication is for, how will it help, how long does it take to work
vi. Concerns about the medication	*'I've taken these tablets in the past they did nothing for me'*
vii. Beliefs towards treatment	Treatment for long term Do not stop when feeling better *'Stops me doing more important things for example driving'*
viii. Choosing not to take medication	30–50% of all people with chronic conditions are non-adherent (Barber 2002) (see Chapter 6)

Table 12.1 summarises these common problems associated with medication. There is a lack of information in the literature relating to the patients' perspective of problems with medication; however, it is clear that many service users have multiple problems related to medication and, as some are resolved, new ones emerge (Barber et al., 2004). It is also important to note that adherence to regular medication regimes are poor, regardless of diagnosis (Vermeire et al., 2001).

i) *Issues associated with health professionals*

Health professionals can cause some difficulties with medication regimes. A common issue is the ability of the service user or case manager to access general practitioners (GPs) or consultant psychiatrists for reviews of medication. Health professionals can also provide inconsistent and differing advice and guidance with regards to medication.

ii and iii)   Practical issues associated with obtaining and taking medication

As highlighted in Table 12.1, there are a number of practical problems associated with the obtaining and taking of medicines. Many of these are self explanatory such as, 'How do you get a repeat prescription?', 'Where is the nearest pharmacist?', 'I can't swallow tablets', 'How can I remember when to take my tablets?' Whilst these examples of practical problems may appear simplistic, they can quickly become insurmountable obstacles to tackle, especially when compounded with a mental health problem. For example, the nearest pharmacist may be two bus journeys away, the service user may have to take the children with him/her, and may be moderately depressed. The process of obtaining a prescription can seem like an ordeal. Alternatively, if service users are on a number of different tablets for both mental and physical health conditions, and the regimes require that they take different tablets four times a day, remembering not only to take the tablets but also which ones to take, can become confusing.

iv)   Effects and side effects of medication

All medication causes side effects, and the side effects associated with psychotropic medication often cause significant problems for service users. For example, weight gain is a particularly problematic side effect, associated with the use of some psychotropic medication. It is proposed that healthcare workers underestimate the problem associated with weight gain and psychotropic medication (Harrison, 2004). Other problems associated with the effects and side effects of psychotropic medication include short-term memory impairments and extra pyramidal side effects (EPSE) such as akathisia. Chapter 2 has detailed the side effects of psychotropic medication in more detail.

People can react badly to psychotropic medication and, paradoxically, some can cause the symptoms they are supposed to treat, for example some of the side effects of antidepressants can be very depressing in themselves. The effects and side effects of commonly prescribed antidepressants include erectile problems, dry mouth, agitation, sleep disruption, nausea, loss of libido and anxiety. In addition to the effects and side effects, issues of dependency and addiction can also become problematic, for example the dependency issues associated with benzodiazepines and some anti-cholinergic medicines such as procyclidine (De Las Cuevas et al., 2003).

v)   Knowledge and information needs

Information needs can potentially cause difficulties for service users, and the poor provision of information regarding medication is well documented. One study identified that service users had needs for further information about medication and about their illness/diagnosis, and the provision of this significantly influenced adherence (Barber et al., 2004).

vi)   Concerns about the medication

Barber and colleagues (2004) discuss how concerns and beliefs about medication are influenced by previous experiences of medication and an individual's illness model. For example, 'I stop taking medication when I feel better', 'I took this pill and it made me feel terrible'.

What is problem solving?

Problem solving is one of many brief psychological interventions that has proven effectiveness as either a single-strand or multi-strand intervention and is widely accepted under the umbrella term of cognitive behavioural therapy (CBT). Problem solving is a systematic way of helping people to manage current difficulties by helping people to feel more in control of their problems and think of more realistic and practical solutions. Problem solving has been defined as:

> 'a behavioural process, whether overt or cognitive in nature, which (a) makes available a variety of potentially effective response alternatives for dealing with the problematic situation and (b) increases the probability of selecting the most effective response from among these various alternatives'
>
> D'Zurilla & Goldfried (1971)

Problem solving is therefore a learning process that helps the decision-making process, and in this sense the application of the problem-solving intervention within medication management is undoubtedly important.

Service users must be encouraged to identify their own problems and solutions and, therefore, the health professional takes a non-directive, supportive stance in the process, promoting service user self management. The essence of problem solving is the generation of solutions to identified problems (Drummond et al., 2005) and a key element is the development of a collaboration partnership between the health professional and the service user.

The history and development of problem solving

D'Zurilla & Goldfried have been attributed with the development of problem solving as a clinical intervention as far back as 1971 (Falloon,

2000a). Their original paper details a five-stage approach to problem solving: general orientation, problem definition, generation of alternatives, decision making and verification (D'Zurilla & Goldfried, 1971). These stages are described in Table 12.2.

D'Zurilla & Goldfried (1971) developed the method from a behavioural perspective, with the initial work conducted with college freshmen before undertaking subsequent testing within mental health institutions. This became the foundations of problem-solving therapy (D'Zurilla & Nezu, 1982).

During the 1970s, the utilisation of problem solving as an intervention was firmly rooted in the field of social work before becoming integrated in clinical trials within mental health research. During the 1980s, problem solving was integrated into CBT and psycho-social interventions (PSI) within the field of psychosis, especially family interventions integrated problem solving as part of a multi-strand intervention package with families. In the 1990s, problem solving was researched within primary care settings, in combination with antidepressant medication. More recently, problem solving has been incorporated into self-help manuals for the treatment of common mental health problems in primary care (Kennedy & Lovell, 2002; Williams, 2002a; Fletcher et al., 2005). An interactive, internet-based version of the *Overcoming Depression* manual is available at www.livinglifetothefull.com by Chris Williams.

Table 12.2 The original five-step approach (adapted from the original text by D'Zurilla & Goldfried, 1971)

Term	Key principles
General orientation	Everyone has problems What is a problem? Think about the problem (no knee-jerk reaction)
Problem definition	Break down (clarify) the problem, make it clear, complete and succinct Rule out the irrelevant
Generation of alternatives	'Brainstorming' (Osborn, 1963) based on four concepts: no wrong answers, the wackier the better, the more the better, merge and improve
Decision-making	Choose the 'best' option
Verification	Determine whether it is the 'best' option, will it solve the problem? Test it out

Evidence base for problem solving

As stated, problem solving has an increasingly robust effectiveness, as either a single-strand or multi-strand intervention, with a range of disorders in both primary and secondary care settings. Within primary care, a number of studies have sought to evaluate the effectiveness of problem solving as a stand-alone intervention and also in combination with antidepressants. There is now evidence of the effectiveness of problem solving with a range of mental health disorders within primary care, regardless of the type of healthcare professional delivering the intervention (Mynors-Wallis, 2002). A Cochrane review of PSIs within primary care highlighted the effectiveness of problem solving as an intervention with major depression (Huibers et al., 2003), although they concluded that more evidence within routine primary care was needed. However, it has been reported that problem solving is no more effective in combination with antidepressants than as a single intervention (Mynors-Wallis et al., 2000). The problem-solving process is now regarded as a stand-alone therapeutic process, 'problem solving therapy' (Nezu & Nezu, 2001).

Within secondary care settings, problem solving has routinely formed part of the family intervention packages, which were successfully undertaken with service users with psychotic disorders and their families (Falloon, 2000). A main feature of psychotic disorders is characterised by difficulties in resolving problems. It is apparent that this remains a need, regardless of the drug therapy an individual receives, and therefore it remains important for clinicians to teach problem-solving skills (Bellack et al., 2004).

The utilisation of problem solving within mental health practice has proven effectiveness, as (Falloon, 2000) concluded:

> *'It may be concluded that problem solving training may be associated with substantial clinical and social benefits for people with major mental health disorders and their key caregivers. These benefits have been observed most clearly in the long-term training of established schizophrenic disorders, but seem to occur with relatively brief applications in the earliest phases of psychotic and affective disorders.'*

Falloon (2000), p. 187

It would seem that this intervention is effective, regardless of the type of health professional delivering it (Mynors-Wallis et al., 1997). However, what remains unclear is whether the application of problem-solving techniques to issues related to medication management will enhance the experiences and adherence to treatment for service users.

The problem-solving process

There are many published variations of the problem-solving process. These range from the original five-step approach (D'Zurilla & Goldfried, 1971) or six (Falloon, 2000) to a seven-step one (Mynors-Wallis, 2002). In order to explain the principles in detail, the version cited within this chapter has been extended to nine steps. Prior to choosing problem solving as the intervention, it is imperative that a thorough assessment of the service user's problem(s) is undertaken. This involves a global style assessment based on the bio-psycho-social model, including assessment of potential risk. Once the assessment has been conducted the service user and the professional collaboratively agree which problem(s) are to be prioritised for treatment.

During the assessment it is also important to identify the resources available to service users, their strengths, supports and assets, to help them overcome their problems, for example close relatives or friends who are aware of the service users' problems and are supportive. This information will help later when working through the steps of problem solving and will make the success of any plans more likely to be positive.

Steps of problem solving

At the beginning of any problem-solving process it is imperative that the health professional explains the rationale and course of the treatment, as well as the benefits that are expected from it. It is also important to emphasise the service user's control of the intervention and the expectation that, once learned, this process can be applied to a plethora of problem situations and that the service user will be able to independently cope with most of these situations.

Step 1: Defining the problem

The need for problem statements to be specific and comprehensive in describing the details of the problem cannot be over-emphasised. Problem statements should be collaboratively agreed between the service user and practitioner to ensure they are service user centred. This is important for a number of factors. Firstly, we have already highlighted that there are numerous reasons why service users become non-adherent with medication, making it imperative that the service user's perspective of the problem is obtained. Secondly, a positive perception of the therapeutic relationship has been found to improve service users' adherence with treatment regimes, improving their outcomes (Holzinger et al., 2002).

Service users rarely present with clear, defined problems and, moreover, their issues are often vague or ambiguous, lacking necessary facts, and much more information is required by the practitioner to ensure that appropriate goals are set for problem solving. It is therefore important to assess the problem thoroughly, gathering information about all the factors involved in the problem. To focus on the problem it can be helpful to use questions which focus on the fourWs (what, where, when and with whom) and ABCs (antecedents, behaviours and cognitions). In defining the problem it is important to ensure that the service user is working with specific problem statements rather than general problems, and it can be useful to begin with open questions and then move onto more closed questions, referred to as the 'funnel sequence' (Kahn & Cannell, 1957). See Figure 12.1 for a diagrammatical version of the funnelling sequence.

Problem statements are usually two to four sentences in length and comprise four key components:

1. the initiating event (trigger, subjective experience)
2. the affective and/or cognitive consequence
3. the behavioural consequence
4. the impact (deficits or excesses).

It is also useful to include information regarding the frequency, intensity or duration of the problem (Lovell et al., 2001). It is worth spending time developing a clear, unambiguous statement, using techniques such as a timeline to obtain an agreed objective description of the problem. The development of such a statement is essential to the process and makes the remaining stages easier.

An example of a general problem might be, 'I do not take my medication', but using specific open questions such as, 'Why do you not take your medication?' followed by closed questions such as, 'How many days in a week do you not take your medication?' helps

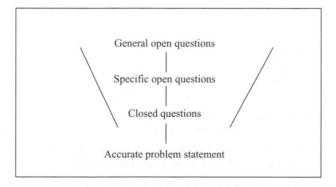

General open questions

Specific open questions

Closed questions

Accurate problem statement

Figure 12.1 Funnel technique for eliciting problem statements.

to establish accurate problem statements. An example of an accurate problem statement might be, 'I forget to take my medication and have only taken 14 out of 28 tablets. Forgetting to take my medication makes me feel low in mood and I start staying in bed which is causing tension between me and my wife.' This is a problem that enables the targeting of solutions and measurement of success.

It can also be useful to rate the level of severity of the problem on a scale of 1–10 where a score of 10 signifies 'this problem troubles me all of the time' and a score of 0 signifies 'this problem does not trouble me at all' as this helps the practitioner to understand how severe the service user rates the problem. Repeating the score at regular intervals during treatment can also help monitor the service user's progress, identifying treatment failures and enabling fast and efficient changes in treatment options and, importantly, providing positive reinforcement for service users by showing that they can, by their own actions, make a difference in what once seemed an intractable problem.

Step 2:   Setting the goal

Goals should be specific, measurable, achievable, realistic and timely (SMART) (Table 12.3).

The best SMART goals are focused and involve things that are under the person's direct control.

Goal statements are usually between one and two sentences in length and comprise four key components (Newell & Gournay, 1999):

1.   the target behaviour/emotion
2.   the setting
3.   the duration
4.   the frequency.

For service users with complex or enduring needs, this may take time to resolve; it may be appropriate to set short-term and long-term goals.

Table 12.3   SMART goals

Specific	Goals should have the expected outcome stated as simply, concisely and explicitly as possible This answers questions such as: how much, for whom, for what?
Measurable	Define objectively how you will know when you have achieved your goal, i.e. an improvement on a scale 1–10
Achievable	An achievable goal has an outcome that is realistic, given your current situation, and the resources and time available
Realistic	Confirm your belief that the goal is indeed possible
Timely	Set a deadline for reaching your goal

Step 3: Ways of achieving the goal (what are the options available to me?)

The next step in the problem-solving process is to brainstorm the options available to service users in helping them to achieve their goal. During this step, service users are encouraged to be inclusive and suggest everything that comes to mind, even if it is unlikely to work. The idea is that the more ideas that are generated, the more likely an option which is likely to help with the problem will be suggested. Evidence suggests that more good ideas are produced under brainstorming instructions than under instructions requesting service users to produce only good ideas (D'Zurilla & Goldfried, 1971). Brainstorming has four basic rules:

- criticism is ruled out – negative judgement of the ideas by the practitioner must be withheld until later;
- 'free-wheeling' is welcome – the wilder the idea, the better;
- quantity is required – the greater the number of ideas, the greater the likelihood of useful ideas;
- combination and improvement are sought – in addition to generating ideas, service users should suggest how ideas of others can be turned into better ideas (What would your friend do in this situation?, How could that work for you?), or how two or more ideas can be joined to improve an idea (Osborn, 1963).

For service users who are struggling to identify options, the practitioner can use questions and provide partial solutions to encourage them to stay focused and not get frustrated by their lack of ideas. A useful technique is to get them to think of what their family and/or friends would suggest for overcoming the problem or what they would suggest to a friend who told them they had a similar problem.

Step 4: List the pros (advantages) and cons (disadvantages) of each option

Despite the generation of possible alternatives, service users are often not able to identify accurately the best of the options they have listed. The process of encouraging critical appraisal is therefore important. In terms of problem solving, the listing of the pros and cons of each of the options identified is a common and useful starting point. A useful question for service users to ask themselves is, 'If I were to carry out this option, what are the various possible consequences, bad and good?'

Step 5: Choosing the most helpful option

Service users then consider each option and its pros and cons and decide on one option that is most likely to help them achieve their goal.

The chosen option should fulfil the following two criteria (Williams, 2002b):

1. Is it helpful?
2. Is it achievable?

Step 6: List the steps needed

Once the most suitable or helpful option has been chosen, the next steps focus on how to plan for the option. It is important for service users to list in a step-by-step fashion exactly what they need to do to achieve the option chosen. It may also be useful for the service user to set achievable timescales for carrying out the necessary steps.

Step 7: Identifying the worse case scenario

Asking the patient about the worse case scenario may help to identify potential barriers that may hinder progress with the problem-solving process (Lever-Green & Hayes, 2008). Any potential barriers can then be discussed to identify how likely it is that the worse case scenario will occur and, where necessary, prepare the service users for any setbacks encountered once they are in the real-life situation of carrying out their treatment. It is often useful to work through some of these issues during treatment so that the person can deal with them more effectively if they do occur.

Step 8: Carry out the chosen option

Step 9: Review outcome

As well as implementing the plan, it is equally important that the outcome of the chosen option is reviewed. Things do not always go as planned and when this happens it is useful to ask questions such as, 'Why did it not work?', 'What could have been done better?'. It maybe necessary to revisit the options listed in Step 3 and the pros and cons in Step 4 to see if another option should be attempted. If you have used the 0–10 rating scale in Step 1, repeat it in the review to establish how much change has occurred. When things do go as planned and people achieve their goals they should be praised for their achievements and also shown how the problem-solving technique may have helped them and how it can be used in other areas of their lives.

An example of how this process can be applied to problems of medication adherence in a primary care setting is now illustrated with a case study (Box 12.1).

Box 12.1 Case study

Problem-solving worksheet			
Step 1	What is the problem?	I forget to take my medication and have only taken 14 out of 28 tablets. Forgetting to take my medication makes me feel low in mood and I start staying in bed, which is causing tension between me and my wife	
Step 2	What are the goals?	I would like to be able to take my medication each day for the next 2 weeks	
Step 3 and 4	What options are there for achieving the goals?	Pros (advantages)	Cons (disadvantages)
	Set an alarm on my watch	I know that it will go off	I might not remember what it is for
	Ask my wife to remind me	Two minds are better than one and therefore twice as likely to remember	She may forget I might over rely on her It might cause more arguments
	Put reminder sticker somewhere I will see it in the morning, i.e. kettle or fridge	I will see it when I get up and it will remind me to take my medication	If I don't get out of bed I won't see sticker
	Have a couple of spare tablets in the car	If I forget in the morning I still have some available during the day	If I don't go in the car it won't help My grandchild might find them
	To take them when I remember	Stops putting pressure on me and making me feel like a failure	I might not get better
Step 5	Which option is most helpful?	Put reminder sticker somewhere I will see it in the morning, i.e. kettle or fridge	
Step 6	What are the steps needed?	Get a packet of post-it notes, write reminder note on some and place one on the kettle, one on the fridge and also one on the bedside cabinet	
Step 7	What is the worse case scenario? Are there any obstacles that might stop/hinder progress?	The shop might have sold out of post-it notes in which case I will use paper and sellotape My wife might move the stickers so I will mention them to her.	
Step 8	Carry out the steps	Step 1: By Monday I will have got some post-it notes Step 2: By Tuesday I will have written them and have them in place	
Step 9	Review (What went well/not so well?)	I remembered to take my medication most days, on 13 out of 14 days, which is a huge improvement Now I want to improve that and not forget it at all in the next 2 weeks	

Figure 12.2 The problem-solving process.

Continued

Bill is a 52-year-old male with a history of moderate depression, which has been ongoing for about a year since being forced to leave work due to ill-health. He has recently been to see his GP, who prescribed an antidepressant and referred him to a primary care mental health worker. Bill has been on the antidepressants for about 4 weeks, but on his first visit describes being forgetful, especially in regards to taking his medication. He has only taken 14 doses of the 28 that he should have had. He believes that they will help him but he cannot seem to remember to take them regularly. The stages of the process are transferred to a problem-solving worksheet to clarify the decisions made and the actions to be taken. There are a number of problem-solving worksheets available for use; an example based on the evidence presented in this chapter is shown in Figure 12.2.

Conclusion

Problem solving is a useful, brief intervention, which is easily mastered by service users and can be used in collaboration with practitioners to aid the medication management process. Using a systematic record of the problem-solving process encourages service users to see alternative solutions to their problems, enables them to think about the pros and cons of each option and, importantly, review the outcome. In reviewing the outcome, service users can be helped to identify the things that went well and the things that did not go as well as expected. As a number of options have been identified the person can easily identify an alternative solution should their first choice prove to be unsuccessful. Importantly, once learned the problem-solving process can be easily applied to other areas of the service user's life. However, it is clear from the limited literature available that further work is required to understand the problems associated with medication from the service users' perspective.

References

Barber, N. (2002) Should we consider non-compliance a medical error? *Quality and Safety in Health Care*, **11**, 81–84.

Barber, N., Parsons, J., Clifford, S., Darracott, R. & Horne, R. (2004) Patients' problems with new medication for chronic conditions. *Quality and Safety in Health Care*, **13**, 172–175.

Bellack, A.S., Schooler, N.R., Marder, S.R., Kane, J.M., Brown, C.H. & Ye Yang, M.S. (2004) Do clozapine and risperidone affect social competence and problem solving? *American Journal of Psychiatry*, **161**, 364–367.

D'Zurilla, T.J. & Goldfried, M.R. (1971) Problem solving and behaviour modification. *Journal of Abnormal Psychology*, **78**, 107–126.

D'Zurilla, T.J. & Nezu, A. (1982) Social problem solving in adults. In: Kendall, P. C. (ed.) *Advances in Cognitive-Behavioural Research and Therapy*. Academic Press, New York.

De Las Cuevas, C., Sanz, E. & De La Fuente, J. (2003) Benzodiazepines: more behavioural addiction than dependence. *Psychopharmacology*, **167**, 297–303.

Drummond, J., Fleming, D., McDonald, L. & Kysela, G. (2005) Randomized controlled trial of family problem-solving intervention. *Clinical Nursing Research*, **14**, 57–80.

Falloon, I.R. (2000) Problem solving as a core strategy in the prevention of schizophrenia and other mental disorders. *Australian and New Zealand Journal of Psychiatry*, **34**(suppl.), S185–S190.

Fletcher, J., Lovell, K., Bower, P. & Campbell, M. (2005) Process and outcome of a non-guided self-help manual for anxiety and depression in primary care: A pilot study. *Behavioural and Cognitive Psychotherapy*, **33**, 319–331.

Harrison, B. (2004) Nursing considerations in psychotropic medication-induced weight gain. *Clinical Nurse Specialist*, **2**, 80–87.

Holzinger, A., Loffler, W., Muller, P., Priebe, S. & Angermeyer, M. (2002) Subjective illness theory and antipsychotic medication compliance by patients with schizophrenia. *Journal of Nervous and Mental Disease*, **190**, 597–603.

Huibers, M.J.H., Beurskens, A.J.H.M., Bleijenberg, G. & Van Schayck, C.P. (2003) *The Effectiveness of Psychosocial Interventions Delivered by General Practitioners*. 2nd edn. The Cochrane Review of Systematic Reviews, York.

Kahn, R.L. & Cannell, C.F. (1957) *The Dynamics of Interviewing: Theory, Technique, and Cases*. Wiley, New York.

Kennedy, A. & Lovell, K. (2002) *A Handy Guide to Managing Depression and Anxiety*. RTFB Publishing Limited, Southampton.

Lever-Green, G. & Hayes, R. (2008) *Skills-based Training on Risk Management (STORM) Participants Handbook*. University of Manchester, Manchester.

Lovell, K., Fox, J. & Bradshaw, T. (2001) What's your problem. *Mental Health & Learning Disabilities Care*, **4**, 377–380.

Mynors-Wallis, L.M. (2002) Does problem solving treatment work through resolving problems? *Psychological Medicine*, **32**, 1315–1319.

Mynors-Wallis, L.M., Gath, D.H., Day, A. & Baker, F. (1997) A randomised controlled trial and cost analysis of problem solving treatment given by community nurses for emotional disorders in primary care. *British Journal of Psychiatry*, **170**, 113–119.

Mynors-Wallis, L.M., Gath, D.H., Day, A. & Baker, F. (2000) Randomised controlled trial of problem solving treatment, antidepressant medication, and combined treatment for major depression in primary care. *British Medical Journal*, **320**, 26–30.

Newell, R. & Gournay, K. (1999) *Mental Health Nursing, an Evidence-based Approach.* Churchill Livingstone, Edinburgh.

Nezu, A. & Nezu, C. (2001) Problem solving therapy. *Journal of Psychotherapy Integration*, **11**, 187–205.

Osborn, A.F. (1963) *Applied Imagination: Principles and Procedures of Creative Problem-solving*, 3rd edn. Scribner's, New York.

Vermeire, E., Hearnshaw, H., Van Royen, P. & Denekens, J. (2001) Patient adherence to treatment: three decades of research: A comprehensive review. *Journal of Clinical Pharmacy and Therapeutics*, **26**, 331–342.

Williams, C. (2002a) *Overcoming Depression.* Arnold Publishers, London.

Williams, C. (2002b) Workbook 2: Practical problem solving. In: Williams, C. (ed.) *Overcoming Depression: A Five Areas Approach.* Arnold Publishing, London.

Key issues for medicines management in inpatient settings

John Baker, Joy Duxbury and Jim Turner

Introduction

Psychotropic medicines are a frequently used and important treatment option in inpatient mental health settings (Bowers et al., 2005). They are routinely seen as the intervention of choice, with most service users admitted to wards receiving them (Paton & Lelliott, 2004). A recent study has estimated that 91% of inpatients were taking two or more medicines for either mental or physical health problems (Healthcare Commission, 2007). A further study of case notes and interviews with 255 inpatients identified restarting medication as the most frequently occurring reason for admission (46%, $n = 117$) (Abas et al., 2003).

This chapter explores some of the medication management issues relevant to inpatient settings. This includes dosage and polypharmacy, the evidence base for dealing with violence and aggression, and service users' experience of medicines in these settings. The chapter then focuses on two specific areas of practice that are underestimated in terms of their importance: the use of *pro re nata* (PRN) psychotropic medication and the safe administration of medicines. It concludes with a case study that highlights a project to change practice associated with the administration of medicines.

Service users' perceptions of medication (in inpatient settings)

The reliance on medication as the dominant treatment option has been criticised by both service users and carers (Johnson et al., 2004; Pollock et al., 2004). Ruane (2004) identified nine anti-therapeutic features of acute mental health wards, three of which relate to medication: firstly, a medication-dominated approach which excludes other forms of therapies, secondly, the side effects of the medication and, thirdly, compulsory treatment. Other factors, such as failure to share decision-making, have emerged as part of the negative experiences associated with treatment, particularly medication (Johnson et al., 2004; Brimblecombe et al., 2007).

Unfortunately, trials and clinical practice rarely reflect the concerns of service users or their preference for oral and single doses of medications, with only a few studies which examine users' views. One study suggested that inpatient service users and staff have a high preference for oral preparations (Müller, 2002). A further study identified a group of service users who were so opposed to having antipsychotic medication that they would prefer physical restraint (Sheline & Nelson, 1993). A recent survey by Gray et al. (2005) of community and inpatient settings identified that about two-thirds of service users were either satisfied or very satisfied with their treatment (68%, $n = 47$) and found medication beneficial (71%, $n = 49$). However, this conflicted with the finding that more than half took medication because they had been told to (54%, $n = 35$). They also experienced side effects (64%, $n = 44$), with 34% of these deemed 'intolerable' ($n = 15$).

Recently, there has been considerable debate about service users and their choices about medication (Perkins & Repper, 1999; Day et al., 2005). Rather than the issue being seen as one of compliance, emphasis should be given to service users making an informed choice about their treatment and care (National Institute of Clinical Excellence, 2002a, 2002b). Lack of information and education about medication and unwanted effects is a consistent theme emerging from user and carer surveys (Howard et al., 2003; Pollock et al., 2004; Ruane, 2004; Gray et al., 2005). Information provision is more likely to occur when new treatments are initiated as it is often assumed that those who have been on treatment for a while know all about them; however, this is often not the case (Happell et al., 2002).

High doses and polypharmacy[1]

The practice of prescribing high doses and/or polypharmacy of antipsychotic medication is not recommended (Harrington et al., 2002a;

[1] Polypharmacy is defined as the use of two or more antipsychotics at the same time. High doses are defined by the *British National Formulary* (*BNF*) limits. High doses in polypharmacy can be calculated either as 'chlorpromazine equivalents' (maximum dose 1000 mg per day) or as percentages of *BNF* limits for each drug added together (Royal College of Psychiatrists, 2006).

Karow & Lambert, 2003; National Institute of Clinical Excellence, 2005; Joint Formulary Committee, 2006). Indeed, one study suggests that long-term exposure to multiple antipsychotic medications leads to premature death (Joukamma et al., 2006). It has been contended that in those individuals with severe symptoms, clinicians may prescribe multiple antipsychotic medications in an attempt to avoid high dose of one particular antipsychotic (Biancosinoa et al., 2005).

A number of UK studies have examined the prevalence of high dose and polypharmacy in antipsychotic prescribing (Warner et al., 1995; Chaplin & McGuigan, 1996; Krasucki & McFarlane, 1996; Newton et al., 1996; Yorston & Pinney, 1997), finding that the prescription of high doses ranged from 2 to 42%. These studies were conducted around the time of the introduction of the Royal College of Psychiatrists consensus statement to prevent high-dose prescribing (Thompson, 1994). A further study, which evaluated the impact of this statement, identified that PRN prescriptions substantially increased the number of service users prescribed high-dose antipsychotics, although only around 5% of these prescriptions were actually used (Milton et al., 1998).

A UK study of 3132 service users in 47 mental health trusts (two-thirds of whom were on acute mental health wards) found 20% (n = 613) were prescribed doses higher than the *British National Formulary* (*BNF*) limit (Harrington et al., 2002a). Prescriptions for PRN antipsychotics accounted for up to half of these potentially high doses. Nearly half (48%, n = 1487) were prescribed more than one antipsychotic. There was considerable variation between services of high doses (range 0 to 50%) and polypharmacy (range 12 to 71%) of antipsychotic medication (Harrington et al., 2002b). The authors speculated that variations in case mix attributed for these differences. Further analysis revealed that age, gender, detention under the *Mental Health Act* and ward setting (rehabilitation and forensic rather than acute) increased antipsychotic polypharmacy, high-dose prescribing and administration (Lelliott et al., 2002). Antipsychotic polypharmacy was found to be the most important factor in causing high doses (Lelliott et al., 2002). These studies used cross-sectional surveys of inpatient populations, which potentially over-estimates the prevalence of both high doses and polypharmacy (Harrington et al., 2002a; Royal College of Psychiatrists, 2006).

Based on these studies, the Royal College of Psychiatry estimates that approximately one quarter of inpatients are prescribed high doses of antipsychotic medication. They attribute these high doses to the effects of polypharmacy, but also suggest that PRN significantly contributes to this (Royal College of Psychiatrists, 2006). However, a recent audit of prescribing practices of acute wards and psychiatric intensive care units (PICUs) in 32 mental health trusts in the UK as part of the

Prescribing Observatory for Mental Health UK (POMH-UK)[2] identified levels higher than the Royal College's estimates for high doses (36%, range 17–71%), multiple antipsychotic medications (43%, range 0–70%) and the co-prescribing of first and second generation antipsychotic medications (31%, range 0–56%) (Healthcare Commission, 2007). Results from the first topic audit cycle suggest that there has been minimal impact on either high doses or polypharmacy prescribing of antipsychotic medication despite a multi-faceted intervention (Paton et al., 2008). The intervention consisted of a clinical workbook (adapted from a previous trial (Thompson et al., 2005)), stickers on prescription cards, posters, workshops and individual feedback to prescribers. Pre–post data from 32 mental health trusts identified that 27% ($n = 945$) of patients were prescribed (or received) high-dose antipsychotics; this compared with 24% ($n = 893$) after the intervention (Paton et al., 2008).

Related literature from studies in emergency psychiatry and comparisons trials for the management of aggression

'On one occasion a patient practised 'Kung fu moves' in the smoking room. A nurse held down his arm and warned that 'if he did not calm down he would be given PRN.'

Ryan and Bowers (2005), p. 697

Trials in emergency psychiatry and comparisons studies of medicines for the management of aggression provide additional information on drugs that are commonly used in inpatient settings. Benzodiazepines (lorazepam, diazepam and midazolam) and antipsychotics (haloperidol, droperidol, olanzapine and ziprasidone) are the most commonly used drugs in these studies. In these trials, drugs have been administered as either single doses or in combinations, aiming to reduce behavioural disturbances, aggression, acute psychosis or mania. There has

[2] POMH-UK was established in March 2005 with Health Foundation funding. It aims to monitor and improve the prescribing of psychotropic medicines in relation to best practice. Seven topics have been identified: i) topic 1, high-dose and combination antipsychotics prescribed on adult acute and psychiatric intensive care wards (PICU) (Oct 2005 to Apr 2007); ii) topic 2, monitoring the physical health of assertive outreach team patients who are prescribed antipsychotics (Oct 2005 to May 2007); iii) topic 3, high-dose and combination antipsychotics prescribed on forensic wards; iv) topic 4, benchmarking antidementia prescribing; v) topic 5, the prescribing of high-dose and combination antipsychotics on adult acute and PICU wards; vi) topic 6, assessment of side effects of antipsychotic drugs in community patients and vii) topic 7, lithium monitoring.

been renewed research interest in this area as older typical antipsychotics (droperidol and thioridazine) have been withdrawn and atypical antipsychotics introduced (De Fruyt & Demyttenaere, 2004).

Acute psychosis

A number of systematic reviews have been conducted on behalf of Cochrane (Waraich et al., 2002;, Carpenter et al., 2004; Gibson et al., 2004; Belgamwar & Fenton, 2005; Gillies et al., 2005) and in other institutions (De Fruyt & Demyttenaere, 2004; Goedhard et al., 2006) of treatments for acute psychosis. The Cochrane reviews have concluded that there is insufficient evidence to support the use of benzodiazepines either alone or in combination with antipsychotic drugs (Gillies et al., 2005) or clotiapine (Carpenter et al., 2004) and zuclopenthixol acetate (Gibson et al., 2004) in acute phases of illness. Although there is some limited evidence for the effectiveness of olanzapine, the authors concluded that this could be seen as ethically biased because of who funded the studies (Belgamwar & Fenton, 2005). Furthermore, the Cochrane review of haloperidol, which is often used as the 'benchmark' treatment, concluded:

> 'It would be understandable, however, if clinicians were cautious in prescribing doses in excess of 7.5 mg/day of haloperidol to a person with uncomplicated acute schizophrenia, and if people with schizophrenia were equally reticent to take greater doses.'
>
> Wariach et al. (2002), pp. 1–2

Another Cochrane review compared combinations of haloperidol plus promethazine for psychosis-induced aggression (Huf et al., 2004) and found that this combination worked better and was safer than using benzodiazepines (lorazepam or midazolam). The authors concluded that trials of these two drugs had randomised the largest total sample of any drug in this area. Despite this finding this combination of drugs is rarely used in the UK.

Violence and aggression

Chemical or physical restraint occurs relatively frequently during an emergency admission (10–20%) (De Fruyt & Demyttenaere, 2004). There is a paucity of research that focuses on clinical interventions for dealing with violence (Department of Health, 2006). This potentially leads to a reliance on pharmacological interventions rather than non-pharmacological ones. A systematic review by Goedhard et al. (2006) examined randomised controlled trials for pharmacological treatment of aggression and failed to identify any strong evidence for its use. In addition, they expressed concerns about flawed study designs and subsequent generalisability of the findings. Particular concerns were general lack of statistical power, trials of too short a duration and a lack of consistency in outcome measurement. They recommended that larger, pragmatic (naturalistic) trials should be undertaken (Goedhard et al., 2006).

A recent UK study identified that PRN medication had the highest approval rating of 11 potential containment methods (Bowers et al., 2004). However, a study in Australia suggested that nurses were more likely to seclude service users than rely on PRN medications (Wynaden et al., 2002), and the authors proposed that this enabled the service user to maintain control, prevent unwanted effects (sedation or disinhibition) and acted as a behavioural intervention. For these staff, seclusion was identified as a safer and less restrictive practice than using PRN medication (Wynaden et al., 2002). In the UK, a study found that medication was a frequent consequence of restraint, occurring 51% ($n = 229$) of the time (Ryan & Bowers, 2006). Forty per cent of those restrained and given medication were given IM medication; although unclear from the published study, these medications were likely to be administered from ongoing PRN prescriptions (C.Ryan, personal communication). Further studies have identified that the use of other behavioural interventions reduces the frequency of assaults, the use of PRN, restraints and seclusion (Donat, 2002a, 2002b, 2005; Bisconer et al., 2006). The use of observations has been found to be highly significant in the reduction of IM medication usage (Damsa et al., 2006).

Rapid tranquilisation[3]

The National Patient Safety Agency has identified four patient safety incidents (PSIs) specific to acute mental health wards. These are: i) absconding, ii) self-harm and suicide, iii) violence (and aggression, including sexual) and iv) harm caused by seclusion, restraint or rapid tranquilisation (National Patient Safety Agency, 2004). Whilst most services have clear policies for rapid tranquilisation based on guidance (National Institute of Clinical Excellence, 2005), the point at which PRN becomes rapid tranquilisation is ambiguous, although it is often

---

[3] Defined as 'the use of medication to calm/lightly sedate the service user, reduce the risk to self and/or others and achieve an optimal reduction in agitation and aggression, thereby allowing a thorough psychiatric evaluation to take place and allowing comprehension and response to spoken messages throughout the intervention. Although not the overt intention, it is recognised that in attempting to calm/lightly sedate the service user, rapid tranquilisation may lead to deep sedation/anaesthesia.' National Institute of Clinical Excellence (2005) p81.

assumed to be the point at which parenteral methods are used (McAllister-Williams & Ferrier, 2002). De Fruyt & Demyttenaere (2004) concluded their systematic review of rapid tranquilisation by suggesting that despite the high frequency of use, they were surprised by the small number of trials conducted in this area. These trials were methodologically flawed in terms of poor design, small samples and varying definitions of rapid tranquilisation, and they failed to report unwanted effects. This, they argued, invalidates the generalisability of the findings. Despite these criticisms, findings from these trials are reflected in some clinical guidelines, with De Fruyt & Demyttenaere (2004) concluding:

> '..in the face of emergency, imminent agitation or aggression where everyone and everyone is out of control, clinicians will stick to personal experience and methods. Hard evidence is needed to challenge and change these "proven habits."'
>
> De Fruyt & Demyttenaere (2004) p. 248

The use of benzodiazepines in inpatient settings

In inpatient settings, benzodiazepines are most commonly used for their sedating properties (Spiegel, 2003). As clinicians have attempted to reduce dependency on older typical antipsychotics, there has been an increased reliance on benzodiazepines, such as lorazapam and diazepam, in acute mental health care (Power et al., 1998; Paton et al., 2000; Richardson & Joseph, 2001). Benzodiazepines are also commonly used as an adjunct to antipsychotic medications (Richardson & Joseph, 2001; Duxbury & Baker, 2004). This contrasts with clinical practice in the community where the use of benzodiazepines has been seen as problematic (Rogers et al., 2007). Lorazepam is often cited as the benzodiazepine drug of choice, especially when IM medication is required, because other benzodiazepines, for example diazepam, have erratic IM absorption (McAllister-Williams & Ferrier, 2002). The use of benzodiazepines in acute mental health wards is widespread. A recent study identified that over 80% of inpatients were prescribed lorazepam during their admission (Choke et al., 2007). However, 40% of the patients never received this, which implies that it was inappropriately prescribed. In a further study, 62% of all drugs given as PRN were benzodiazepines; lorazepam accounted for over half of all drugs given (Baker et al., 2008a). There are a range of side effects associated with their use, most notably rebound anxiety or insomnia, disturbed behaviour and, in severe cases, respiratory depression and toxicity (with long half-life drugs) (Stahl, 2000; Spiegel, 2003); further information on these have been provided in earlier chapters.

PRN psychotropic medication

> *'Our findings indicate that the use of PRN orders may expose psychiatric inservice users to unnecessary psychotropic medications. Given the objective of regulatory bodies to minimise the use of 'chemical restraints' in the population of vulnerable patients, these findings have important policy implications.'*
>
> *Thapa et al. (2003), p. 1286*

PRN psychotropic medications are a frequently used clinical intervention in inpatient settings. Approximately 80% of patients are likely to receive PRN psychotropic medications whilst inpatients (Geffen et al., 2002; Curtis and Capp, 2003). Patients are most likely to receive them early in an admission, although a small group continue to receive a high number of PRN administrations throughout the admission (Vitiello et al., 1987; McLaren et al., 1990; McKenzie et al., 1999; Usher et al., 2001; Geffen et al., 2002; Curtis & Capp, 2003; Thapa et al., 2003). Administration of PRN medication is most likely to occur during the evening (Bernard & Littlejohn, 2000; Stratton-Powell, 2001; Usher et al., 2001). Benzodiazepines, antipsychotics, hypnotics and antihistamines are most likely to be used (Blair & Ramones, 1998; McKenzie et al., 1999).

In a recent literature review, several issues emerged which clinical staff and researchers need to consider further to enhance practice in this area (Baker et al., 2008b). Firstly, the routine prescribing of PRN allows the administration of PRN early in a patient's admission, when little is known about the patient. Secondly, PRN continues to be prescribed and administered for complex phenomena such as agitation. Thirdly, there is a continued reliance on typical antipsychotic medications for use as PRN; this undoubtedly contributes to polypharmacy and high doses. A recent study attempted to improve the manner in which PRN psychotropic medications were used. It employed a two-phase design based on the Medical Research Council's complex intervention framework. The first phase developed a good practice manual. Four studies contributed to this, which included a literature review (best-evidence synthesis), interviews with the multi-disciplinary team ($n = 59$) and service users ($n = 22$), and a Delphi study with experts ($n = 18$) (Baker et al., 2006a, 2006b, 2007, 2008b). The second phase used a pre–post test design to undertake an exploratory and acceptability trial of the manual (Baker et al., 2008a). The contents of the manual (nine themes of good practice) were based on these findings. Recommendations included:

- consideration should be given to the patient knowledge, preferences and choices of medications;
- improving the quality of prescriptions for PRN medication;

- PRN should be part of the clinical management plan;
- the effects and side effects of PRN should be evaluated;
- PRN should be frequently reviewed;
- documentation associated with the prescribing and administration of PRN by the multi-disciplinary team should be enhanced, e.g. recording when PRN has been administered, the rationale for giving as well as effects and side effects experienced;
- distress associated with PRN should be prevented, e.g. by increasing privacy at times of administration, negotiation were possible;
- PRN should be used as a last resort, and the use of alternative non-pharmacological interventions encouraged;
- additional training and education on psychotropic medication and PRN is required for all clinical staff.

In phase two (the exploratory and acceptability trial), 28 of 35 patients received 484 doses of PRN in the 10-week period. Patients had a mean of 3.6 prescriptions of 14 different PRN medications in 34 different dose combinations prescribed. Medication errors beyond poor quality of prescribing occurred in 23 of the 35 patients (66%). Prescription quality improved following the introduction of the intervention but quality of nursing notes reduced. Acceptability of the manual to both nursing and medical staff was high (Baker et al., 2008a).

The administration of medication

Psychotropic medication is widely recognised as a key component of many inpatient admissions. It remains largely the responsibility of registered nurses to administer prescribed medication (Haglund et al., 2004). Consequently, the Nursing and Midwifery Council (NMC) (2008) continue to revisit standards to guide practitioners in this complex task. This includes the need to provide education about the medication, including its effectiveness and side effects (Gray et al., 2002; Baker et al., 2006a; Nursing and Midwifery Council, 2008). In undertaking this procedure, nurses are required to make judgements regarding service users' mental capacity (Forsyth, 2007) and to employ a range of skills in therapeutic communication (Olofsson et al., 1999).

It has been suggested that the administration of medication may be 'the highest risk task a nurse can perform' (Anderson & Webster, 2001). Despite this, research has identified that nursing staff may have a poor knowledge base, be inexperienced, and feel 'stressed' about and have inadequate supervision and support with regards to the administration of medication (Grant & Townsend, 2007; Schelbred and Nord, 2007). These factors may contribute to the increasing incidence of the misadministration of medication (Stubbs et al., 2006).

The Department of Health (2004) estimates that there is a 5% error rate in the administration of medicines in hospitals, and that it harms 1–2% of admitted patients (Maidment et al., 2006). Heavy workloads and increasing numbers and dosages of medicines prescribed presents hard-pressed staff with a challenge when endeavouring to complete this task efficiently.

Factors such as these also affect the service users' acceptance of medication and their subsequent decision to adhere to the long-term use of psychotropic medication. For example, Day et al. (2005) found that patients' experience of admission and interactions with staff significantly impacted upon their adherence with medication. Further research into aspects of medicines management in inpatient settings is clearly required, in particular a greater understanding of the experience of both giving and receiving medication in this setting.

Four key areas are of particular importance when administering medication in the acute inpatient environment: the procedure, monitoring of effectiveness, provision of information and therapeutic engagement.

The procedure

Issues relating to the administration of medication account for nearly a quarter (22%) of the time nurses are in contact with service users, and nearly 10% of their total time (data collected between 7am and 6pm) (Whittington & McLaughlin, 2000). Practices with regard to the administration of medication and medication rounds, however, are variable in the UK. The use of medication trolleys and 'gates' continue to feature as common approaches, despite the evidence that they are responsible for medication error and the benefits of self-administration. Medication errors during medication rounds are often attributed to poor, careless nursing practice, commonly believed to be the result of stressful nursing environments (Dickens, 2007; Schelbred & Nord, 2007). This is further compounded by the interruptions and distractions that occur simultaneously and that contribute to the stressful and chaotic nature of many ward environments (Manias et al., 2004).

The multifaceted role of the nurse, to simultaneously ensure correct identity, assess the service user's condition, the effects and side effects of medication, and maintain clear and accurate records, contributes to the pressures associated with this complex procedure (Nursing and Midwifery Council, 2008). Noisy and busy environments and tired and overstretched nurses can have an effect upon the nurses' perspective, if not their performance (Haw et al., 2005). Procedures for the administration of medication in acute inpatient areas therefore warrant greater consideration, particularly with regard to design and execution.

Monitoring of effectiveness

Information gathering when making judgements about medication administration is essential. Effective monitoring in acute mental health settings, however, is reportedly scarce (Richards et al., 2005). It is in fact suggested that healthcare workers underestimate the problems associated with side effects and psychotropic medication (Harrison, 2004). Higgins et al. (2006) argues that the nurse's role in assessing the therapeutic and non-therapeutic effects of medication is non-negotiable. Time constraints and the nurse's lack of knowledge are blamed most commonly for deficiencies in practice (Higgins et al., 2006; Castledine, 2007).

Provision of information

Information needs to be provided in both written and oral formats (Healthcare Commission, 2007). Although research suggests new service users are provided with information, it is often assumed that those who have been on treatment for some time know all about it; this is often not the case (Happell et al., 2002). Information provided should be clear, brief, repetitive, ongoing and accurate, detailing the medication prescribed. The process also needs to include the service user in the decision-making process (Happell et al., 2004; Janssen et al., 2006). Accurate record keeping and communication regarding matters of this sort is a key directive in the new NMC standards (Nursing and Midwifery Council, 2008).

Therapeutic engagement

If the service users' perception of inpatient services is positive, including a non-coercive atmosphere, positive relationships with the care team, a regimen with minimal adverse effects and involvement in treatment decisions, they are more prepared to accept treatment (Day et al., 2005). The establishment of a therapeutic relationship is pivotal to enhancing medication adherence (Pollock et al., 2004; Gray et al., 2005,). It is through positive engagement that a climate of trust can be created where patients feel able to disclose their thoughts about the potential impact of medication (Higgins et al., 2006). Haglund et al. (2004) describe the frustration that service users experience when there is a lack of interpersonal contact during medication administration and see this as a missed opportunity to communicate with nurses (p. 233). A good working alliance between service users and nurses, which respects and values their views, can re-establish engagement with treatment and ultimately lead to the development of self-efficacy in medication management (Usher & Arthur, 1998; Day et al., 2005).

A case study on managing change in medication administration is given in Box 13.1.

Box 13.1   Case study – Managing change in medication administration

Concern was expressed by a stakeholder group of clients, relatives and staff about the administration of medicines in a large, inner city, acute inpatient service. It was decided that a change strategy was needed to ensure consistent standards of medication administration across all the wards at the same time period. It is generally accepted that standards help improve the quality of care (Johns, 1990). A service improvement project was therefore developed to address these concerns (Turner et al., 2007, 2008). Two stages were agreed upon by the leaders of the project.

Stage 1:   Development and implementation of a structured assessment for the administration of patient medicines

Ito & Syun (2003) have identified problems with the medication round, including:

- it is an inefficient use of time, often requires two nurses and so the workload of others increases to compensate for this
- drugs are not always given at the correct time
- relatives and service users are passive in the process with little time for explanation
- the value of the round as a teaching tool remains unclear as students are often used to guard the trolley.

The project aimed to:

1. develop a standard assessment for the administration of medicines
2. help move towards individual patient administration and the associated educational aspects inherent within an individual administration.

The medicines assessment was designed to improve administration practice, increase service user involvement in their medicines and facilitate compliance with medication through active engagement in the process of medicines management early on in the care. We were concerned about the usual hospital procedures of drug rounds, polypharmacy, fixed medication regimens and a staff-led medicines organisation, which did not necessarily mirror the service users' daily routines. We were also aware of issues of breaches to confidentiality when queues formed at medication time.

The medication assessment was based upon a review of the literature and incorporated both an assessment and a set of clinical guidelines, following the format of the Maudsley (Ritter, 1993) and Royal Marsden (Dougherty & Lister, 2004) clinical procedures. Assessments were initially undertaken in the peer group to facilitate reliability and application of the assessment tool, later used for preceptorship and student nurses. There are 37 assessed aspects of a drug administration and management procedure, which encompass environmental, preparation, administration and housekeeping activities. There are also nine multi-choice questions assessing medication knowledge (including effects and side effects).

All staff were supported in the adoption of the 'standard' by the ward managers and the project team, the service user representative being integral to this process. Staff had to 'pass' the assessment within the project timescale. Systems were put in place to support staff who required further development; this was potentially a difficult situation as these staff were already working clinically. The vehicle for change was, therefore, to ensure staff were familiar with the assessment to enable them to be 'assessors' of students on placement. With this approach all staff were provided with the expected standard.

Stage 2

Hughes et al. (1997) suggest treatment protocols should be organised around the individual requirements and lifestyle, but to get to this one has to first provide adequate information about the effects and side effects of medications, both when the individual is ill and he or she is getting better. A medicines management programme, based upon a health belief rather than a medical model of care, was therefore developed. The plan was to develop individual nursing practice to a level where an individual's understanding of medicines would enable service users to make reasonable decisions about the benefits of taking medicines. The aims were to:

1. develop and evaluate a social model of adherence
2. provide structured medication information, giving sessions on the wards
3. develop support structures for people on medicines, based on a knowledgeable position rather than one lacking in awareness
4. move toward a position where all administration is carried out individually and not from a trolley or cupboard where a queue could form.

The skills programme involved 2 weeks of intensive training for two staff nurses from each of the inpatient wards. Six main areas were included in the taught sessions, which were delivered by the project leads, suitably qualified staff and service users. Service users were integral to the whole process of the project and their sessions included talking from their own experience about their medication management needs and issues. Staff returned to their wards following the training and were supported with a practice manual and regular supervision. Supervision emphasised the importance of continuous knowledge and skills development. Positive outcomes were achieved in a number of areas, with some slippage in others.

Continued

In achieving change we were mindful of work undertaken into understanding the emotional state of organisations as it is well recognised that emotional processes can enhance the study of organisations (Walsh, 1996). A process of project management and change management, combined with pragmatic recognition of the limitations and steps normally taken in the change process, was applied. Individuals have different levels of motivation for change and, for some, to have resistance (Dallos & Vetere, 2005), hence our strategy was to use both change models and the 'authority' in the Trust hierarchy as leverage. Our approach was guided by the cognitive model described by Prochaska & DiClemente (1982). This model suggests that, for change to happen, individuals have to take steps of pre-contemplation, contemplation (self and others), preparation and action. Although this model is well rounded, we also drew upon models which have 'energy' as their lever, such as 'change management' guidance from popular management manuals' for example *Who Moved my Cheese?* (Johnson, 1998), more recently updated and discussed in *FISH!* (Lundin et al., 2002) and *Our Iceberg is Melting* (Kotter, 2005). Johnson (1998) and Kotter (2005) share similar positions, suggesting that a number of factors are important to encourage change in organisations. These factors primarily focus on adapting to change, generating energy for change, monitoring change, valuing the organisational culture when changing and changing the culture, and making change continue . . . making it stick.

Conclusion

There is substantial evidence for the use of both antipsychotics and benzodiazepines in inpatient settings. They are a frequently used intervention in acute mental health wards for a range of reasons, including psychosis and behavioural disturbances. However, the use of medication is frequently criticised as being the only treatment option in inpatient care. Information provision and choice by service users is often neglected. This chapter has highlighted some important aspects of medicines management in inpatient settings, particularly the continued use of high doses and polypharmacy of antipsychotic medication. The role of PRN contributes to this problem. It also highlights issues associated with the administration of medicines in these settings.

Acknowledgements

We acknowledge support from the Health Foundation, who supported the research into PRN psychotropic medication with a Nursing and Allied Health Professions Training Fellowship.

The Burdett Trust for Nursing supported the research into the administration of medicines.

References

Abas, M., Vanderpyl, J., LeProu, T., Kydd, R., Emery, B. & Foliaki, S. (2003) Psychiatric hospitalisation: reasons for admission and alternatives to admission in South Auckland, New Zealand. *Australian and New Zealand Journal of Psychiatry*, **37**, 620–625.

Anderson, D. & Webster, C. (2001) A systems approach to the reduction of medication error on the hospital ward. *Journal of Advanced Nursing*, **35**(1), 34–41.

Baker, J., Lovell, K. & Harris, N. (2008a) The impact of good practice guidelines on professional practice associated with psychotropic PRN in acute mental health wards: An exploratory study. *International Journal of Nursing Studies*, **45**, 1403–1410. doi: 10.1016/j.ijnurstu.2008.01.004.

Baker, J.A., Lovell, K. & Harris, N. (2006b) How expert are the experts: an exploration of the concept of expert within Delphi panel techniques. *Nurse Researcher*, **14**(1), 59–70.

Baker, J.A., Lovell, K. & Harris, N. (2007) Mental health professionals' psychotropic pro re nata (p.r.n.) medication practices in acute inpatient mental health care: a qualitative study. *General Hospital Psychiatry*, **29**, 163–168.

Baker, J.A., Lovell, K. & Harris, N. (2008b) The administration of psychotropic pro re nata (PRN) medication in inpatient mental health settings: a best-evidence synthesis review. *Journal of Clinical Nursing*, **17**(9), 1122–1131.

Baker, J.A., Lovell, K., Easton, K. & Harris, N. (2006a) Service users' experiences of 'as needed' psychotropic medications in acute mental healthcare settings. *Journal of Advanced Nursing*, **56**(4), 1–9.

Belgamwar, R.B. & Fenton, M. (2005) Olanzapine IM or velotab for acutely disturbed/agitated people with suspected serious mental illnesses (review). In: *Cochrane Database of Systematic Reviews (2) Art. No.: CD003729*.

Bernard, P. & Littlejohn, R. (2000) The use of 'as required' medication on an adolescent psychiatric unit. *Clinical Child Psychology and Psychiatry*, **5**(2), 258–266.

Biancosinoa, B., Barbuic, C., Marmaia, L., Dona, S. & Grassia, L. (2005) Determinants of antipsychotic polypharmacy in psychiatric inpatients: a prospective study. *International Clinical Psychopharmacology*, **20**, 305–309.

Bisconer, S., Green, M., Mallon-Czajka, J. & Johnson, J. (2006) Managing aggression in a psychiatric hospital using a behaviour plan: a case study. *Journal of Psychiatric and Mental Health Nursing*, **13**, 515–521.

Blair, T. & Ramones, V. (1998) Understanding PRN medications in psychiatric care. *Perspectives*, **3**(2).

Bowers, L., Alexander, J., Simpson, A., Ryan, C. & Carr-Walker, P. (2004) Cultures of psychiatry and the professional socialization process: the case of containment methods for disturbed patients. *Nurse Education Today*, **24**, 435–442.

Bowers, L., Simpson, A., Alexander, J., et al. (2005) The nature and purpose of acute psychiatric wards: the Tompkins Acute Ward Study. *Journal of Mental Health*, **14**(6), 625–635.

Brimblecombe, N., Tingle, A. & Murrells, T. (2007) How mental health nursing can best improve service users' experiences and outcomes in inpatient settings: responses to a national consultation. *Journal of Psychiatric & Mental Health Nursing*, **14**, 503–509.

Carpenter, S., Berk, M. & Rathbone, J. (2004) Clotiapine for acute psychotic illnesses (review). In: *Cochrane Database of Systematic Reviews, (2) Art. No.: CD001951*, Vol. 3.

Castledine, G. (2007) Perils of the drug round. *British Journal of Nursing*, **16**(17), 1101.

Chaplin, R. & McGuigan, S. (1996) Antipsychotic dose: from research to clinical practice. *Psychiatric Bulletin*, **20**, 452–454.

Choke, A., Perumal, M. & Howlett, M. (2007) Lorazepam prescription and monitoring in acute psychiatric wards. *Psychiatric Bulletin*, **31**, 300–303.

Curtis, J. & Capp, K. (2003) Administration of 'as needed' psychotropic medication: a retrospective study. *International Journal of Mental Health Nursing*, **12**, 229–234.

Dallos, R. & Vetere, A. (2005) *Researching Psychotherapy and Counselling*. Open University Press, London.

Damsa, C., Ikelheimer, D., Adam, E., et al. (2006) Heisenberg in the ER: observation appears to reduce involuntary intramuscular injections in a psychiatric emergency setting. *General Hospital Psychiatry*, **28**(5), 431–433.

Day, J., Bentall, R., Roberts, C., et al. (2005) Attitude toward antipsychotic medication: the impact of clinical variables and relationships with health professionals. *Archives of General Psychiatry*, **62**, 717–724.

De Fruyt, J. & Demyttenaere, K. (2004) Rapid tranquilization: new approaches in the emergency treatment of behavioural disturbances. *European Psychiatry*, **19**(5), 243–249.

Department of Health (2004) *Building a safer NHS for patients: improving medication safety.* Department of Health, London.

Department of Health (2006) *From value to actions: The Chief Nursing Officer's review of mental health nursing*. Department of Health, London.

Dickens, G. (2007) Inpatient psychiatry: three methods to detect medication errors. *Nurse Prescribing*, **4**(4), 167–171.

Donat, D. (2002a) Employing behavioral methods to improve the context of care in a public psychiatric hospital: reducing hospital reliance on seclusion/restraint and psychotropic PRN medication. *Cognitive and Behavioral Practice*, **9**(1), 28–37.

Donat, D. (2002b) Impact of improved staffing on seclusion/restraint reliance in a public psychiatric hospital. *Psychiatric Rehabilitation Journal*, **25**(4), 413–416.

Donat, D. (2005) Encouraging alternatives to seclusion, restraint, and reliance on PRN drugs in public psychiatric hospital. *Psychiatric Services*, **56**(9), 1105–1108.

Dougherty, L. & Lister, S. (2004) *The Royal Marsden Hospital Manual of Clinical Nursing Procedures*, 6th edn. Royal Marsden NHS Trust and Blackwells, London.

Duxbury, J. & Baker, J.A. (2004) The use and nursing management of benzodiazepines in acute, mental health inpatient care: a discussion. *Journal of Psychiatric and Mental Health Nursing*, **11**, 662–667.

Forsyth, L. (2007) The Mental Capacity Act: what you need to know. *Mental Health Practice*, **11**(1), 16–19.y

Geffen, J., Sorensen, L., Stokes, J., Cameron, A., Roberts, M.S. & Geffen, L. (2002) Pro re nata medication for psychoses: an audit of practice in two metropolitan hospitals. *Australian and New Zealand Journal of Psychiatry*, **36**, 649–656.

Gibson, R.C., Fenton, M., Coutinho, E.S. & Campbell, C. (2004) Zuclopenthixol acetate for acute schizophrenia and similar serious mental illnesses (review). In: *Cochrane Database of Systematic Reviews. (3): Art. No.: CD000525.y*

Gillies, D., Beck, A., McCloud, A. & Rathbone, J. (2005) Benzodiazepines alone or in combination with antipsychotic drugs for acute psychosis (review). In: *Cochrane Database of Systematic Reviews, (4) Art. No.: CD003079.*

Goedhard, L., Stollker, J., Heerdink, E., Nijman, H., Olivier, B. & Egberts, A. (2006) Pharmacotherapy for the treatment of aggressive behaviour in general adult psychiatry: A systematic review. *Journal of Clinical Psychiatry*, **67**(7), 1013–1024.

Grant, A. & Townsend, M. (2007) Some emerging implications for clinical supervision in British mental health nursing. *Journal of Psychiatric and Mental Health Nursing*, **14**, 609–614.

Gray, R., Rofail, D., Allen, J. & Newey, T. (2005) A survey of patient satisfaction with and subjective experience of treatment with antipsychotic medication. *Journal of Advanced Nursing*, **52**(1), 31–37.

Gray, R., Wykes, T. & Gournay, K. (2002) From compliance to concordance: a review of the literature to enhance compliance with antipsychotic medication. *Journal of Psychiatric and Mental Health Nursing*, **9**, 277–284.

Haglund, K., Von-Essen, L. & Von Knorring, L. (2004) Medication administration in inpatient psychiatric care – get control and leave control. *Journal of Psychiatric & Mental Health Nursing.* **11**, 229–234.

Happell, B., Manias, E. & Pinikahana, J. (2002) The role of the inpatient mental health nurse in facilitating patient adherence to medication regimes. *International Journal of Mental Health Nursing,* **11**, 251–259.

Happell, B., Manias, E. & Roper, C. (2004) Wanting to be heard: mental health consumers' experiences of information about medication. *International Journal of Mental Health Nursing,* **13**, 242–248.

Harrington, M., Lelliott, P., Paton, C., Konsolaki, M., Sensky, T. & Okocha, C. (2002a) Variations between services in polypharmacy and combined high dose of antipsychotic drugs prescribed for in-patients. *Psychiatric Bulletin,* **26**, 418–420.

Harrington, M., Lelliott, P., Paton, C., Okocha, C., Duffett, R. & Sensky, T. (2002b) The results of a multi-centre audit of the prescribing of antipsychotic drugs for in-patients in the UK. *Psychiatric Bulletin,* **26**, 414–418.

Harrison, B. (2004) Nursing considerations in psychotropic medication-induced weight gain. *Clinical Nurse Specialist,* **2**(18), 80–87.

Haw, C.M., Dickens, G. & Stubbs, J. (2005) A review of medication errors reported in a large psychiatric hospital in the United Kingdom. *Psychiatric Services,* **56**(12), 1610–1613.

Healthcare Commission (2007) *talking about medicines. the management of medicines in trusts providing mental health services.* Commission for Healthcare Audit and Inspection, London.

Higgins, A., Barker, P. & Begley, C.M. (2006) Iatrogenic sexual dysfunction and withholding of information. *Journal of Psychiatric and Mental Health Nursing,* **13**, 437–446.

Howard, P., El-Mallakh, P., Rayens, M. & Clark, J. (2003) Consumer perspectives on quality of inpatient mental health services. *Archives of Psychiatric Nursing,* **17**(5), 205–215.

Huf, G., Alexander, J. & Allen, M. (2004) Haloperidol plus promethazine for psychosis induced aggression. In: *Cochrane Database of Systematic Reviews: Issue 4 Art. No.: CD005146.*

Hughes, I., Hill, B. & Budd, R. (1997) Compliance with antipsychotic medication: From theory to practice. *Journal of Mental Health,* **6**(5), 473–489.

Ito, H. & Syun, Y. (2003) Common types of medication errors on long-term psychiatric units. *International Journal for Quality in Healthcare,* **15**(3), 207–212.

Johns, C. (1990) Steps to self medication. *Nursing Times,* **86**(11), 40–41.

Johnson, S. (1998) *Who Moved My Cheese? An Amazing Way to Deal with Change in Your Work and in Your Life.* Putnam Publications Group, New York.

Johnson, S., Bingham, C., Billings, J., et al. (2004) Women's experiences of admission to a crisis house and to acute hospital wards: a qualitative study. *Journal of Mental Health,* **13**(3), 247–262.

Joint Formulary Committee (2006) *British National Formulary.* British Medical Association and Royal Pharmaceutical Society of Great Britain, London.

Joukamma, M., Heliovaara, M., Knekt, P., Aromaa, A., Raitasalo, R. & Lehtinen, V. (2006) Schizophrenia, neuroleptic medication and mortality. *British Journal of Psychiatry,* **188**, 122–127.

Karow, A. & Lambert, M. (2003) Polypharmacy in treatment with psychotropic drugs: The underestimated phenomenon. *Current Opinion in Psychiatry,* **16**, 713–718.

Kotter, J. (2005) *Our Iceberg is Melting: Changing and Succeeding Under Any Conditions.* Macmillan, Washington.

Krasucki, C. & McFarlane, F. (1996) Electrocardiograms, high-dose antipsychotic treatment and colleague guidelines. *Psychiatric Bulletin,* **20**, 326–330.y

Lelliott, P., Paton, C., Harrington, M., Konsolaki, M., Sensky, T. & Okocha, C. (2002) The influence of patient variables on polypharmacy and combined high dose of antipsychotic drugs prescribed for in-patients. *Psychiatric Bulletin,* **26**, 411–414.

Lundin, S., Paul, H. & Christensen, J. (2002) *"FISH!" A Remarkable Way to Boost Morale and Improve Results.* Hyperion Publishers, New York.

Maidment, I., Lelliott, P. & Paton, C. (2006) Medication errors in mental healthcare: A systematic review. *Quality and Safety in Health Care,* **15**, 409–413.

Manias, E., Aitken, R. & Dunning, T. (2004) Medication management by graduate nurses: Before, during and following medication administration. *Nursing & Health Sciences,* **6**(2), 83–91.

McAllister-Williams, H. & Ferrier, N. (2002) Rapid tranquillisation: time for a reappraisal of options for parenteral therapy. *British Journal of Psychiatry,* **180**, 485–489.

McKenzie, A., Kudinoff, T., Benson, A. & Archillingham, A. (1999) Administration of PRN medication: a descriptive study of nursing practice. *Australian & New Zealand Journal of Mental Health Nursing,* **8**(4), 187–191.

McLaren, S., Browne, F. & Taylor, P. (1990) A study of psychotropic medication given 'As required' in a Regional Secure Unit. *British Journal of Psychiatry,* **156**, 732–735.

Milton, J., Lawton, J., Smith, M. & Buckley, A. (1998) Hidden high-dose antipsychotic prescribing: Effects of PRN doses. *Psychiatric Bulletin,* **22**(11), 675–677.

Müller, M.J. (2002) Patients' satisfaction with psychiatric treatment: comparison between an open and a closed ward. *Psychiatric Quarterly,* **73**(2), 93–107.

National Institute of Clinical Excellence (2002a) *Guidance on the use of newer (atypical) antipsychotic drugs for the treatment of schizophrenia.* Department of Health, London.

National Institute of Clinical Excellence (2002b) *Schizophrenia: Core interventions in the treatment and management of schizophrenia in primary and secondary care.* Department of Health, London.

National Institute of Clinical Excellence (2005) *Violence: the short-term management of disturbed/violent behaviour in in-patient psychiatric settings and emergency departments.* Department of Health, London.

National Patient Safety Agency (2004) *Safer wards for acute psychiatry. a review of the available evidence.* Department of Health, London.

Newton, K., Murthy, R. & Qureshi, J. (1996) Antipsychotic prescribing in light of the consensus statement of the college. *Psychiatric Bulletin*, **21**, 408–410.

Nursing and Midwifery Council (2008) *Standards for Medicines Management.* Nursing and Midwifery Council, London.

Olofsson, B., Jacobsson, L., Gilje, F. & Norberg, A. (1999) Being in conflict: Physicians' experience with using coercion in psychiatric care. *Nordic Journal of Psychiatry*, **5**, 203–210.

Paton, C. & Lelliott, P. (2004) The use of prescribing indicators to measure quality of care in psychiatric inpatients. *Quality and Safety in Health Care*, **13**, 40–45.

Paton, C., Banham, S. & Whitmore, J. (2000) Benzodiazepines in schizophrenia: Is there a trend towards long-term prescribing? *Psychiatric Bulletin*, **24**, 113–115.

Paton, C., Barnes, T., Cavanagh, M., Taylor, D. & Lelliott, P. (2008) High-dose and combination antipsychotic prescribing in acute adult wards in the UK: The challenges posed by p.r.n. prescribing. *British Journal of Psychiatry*, **192**, 435–439.

Perkins, J. & Repper, J. (1999) Compliance or informed choice. *Journal of Mental Health*, **8**(2), 117–129.

Pollock, K., Grime, J., Baker, E. & Mantala, K. (2004) Meeting the information needs of psychiatric inpatients: Staff and patient perspectives. *Journal of Mental Health*, **13**(4), 389–401.

Power, P., Elkins, K., Adlard, S., Curry, C., McGorry, P. & Harrigan, S. (1998) Analysis of the initial treatment phase in first-episode psychosis. *British Journal of Psychiatry*, **172**(Suppl. 33), 71–76.

Prochaska, J.O. & DiClemente, C.C. (1982) Transtheoretical therapy: Towards a more integrative model of change. *Psychotherapy, Theory, Research and Practice*, **20**, 161–73.

Richards, D., Bee, P., Loftus, S.J., Baker, J.A., Bailey, L. & Lovell, K. (2005) Specialist educational intervention for acute inpatient mental health nursing staff: service user views and effects on nursing quality. *Journal of Advanced Nursing*, **51**(6), 634–644.

Richardson, J.P. & Joseph, S. (2001) Antipsychotics in acute agitation. *Psychiatric Bulletin*, **25**, 276–7.

Ritter, S. (1993) *Bethlem Royal and Maudsley Hospital: Manual of Clinical Psychiatric Nursing Principles and Procedures.* Chapman and Hall, London.

Rogers, A., Pilgrim, D., Brennan, S., Sulaiman, I., Watson, G. & Chew-Graham, C. (2007) Prescribing benzodiazepines in general practice: a new view of an old problem. *Health: An Interdisciplinary Journal for the Social Study of Health, Illness and Medicine*, **11**(2), 181–198.

Royal College of Psychiatrists. (2006) *Consensus statement on high-dose antipsychotic medication.* Royal College of Psychiatrists, London.

Ruane, P. (2004) A carer's perception of the therapeutic value of in-patient settings. In: Campling, P., Davis, S. & Farquharson, G.) *From Toxic Institutions to Therapeutic Environments. Residential Settings in Mental Health Services.* pp. 166–173. Gaskell, London,.

Ryan, C. & Bowers, L. (2006) An analysis of nurses' post-incident manual restraint reports. *Journal of Psychiatric and Mental Health Nursing*, **13**, 527–532.

Ryan, C.J. & Bowers, L. (2005) Coercive manoeuvres in a psychiatric intensive care unit. *Journal of Psychiatric and Mental Health Nursing*, **12**, 695–702.

Schelbred, A.B. & Nord, R. (2007) Nurses' experiences of drug administration errors. *Journal of Advanced Nursing*, **60**(3), 317–324.

Sheline, Y. & Nelson, T. (1993) Patient choice: deciding between psychotropic medication and physical restraints in an emergency. *Bulletin of the American Academy of Psychiatry and the Law*, **21**(3), 321–329.

Spiegel, R. (2003) *Psychopharmacology: An Introduction.* John Wiley & Sons Ltd., Chichester.

Stahl, S. (2000) *Essential Psychopharmacology. Neuroscientific Basis and Practical Applications.* Cambridge University Press, Cambridge.

Stratton-Powell, H. (2001) *PRN lorazepam: The nurse's judgement, the nurse's decision.* Master of Philosophy, The School of Nursing, Midwifery and Social Work, The University of Manchester, Manchester.

Stubbs, J., Haw, C. & Taylor, D. (2006) Prescription errors in psychiatry – a multi-centre study. *Journal of Psychopharmacology*, **20**(4), 553–561.

Thapa, P., Palmer, S., Huntley, A., Clardy, J. & Miller, L. (2003) PRN (as needed) orders and exposure of psychiatric inpatients to unnecessary psychotropic medications. *Psychiatric Services*, **54**(9), 1282–1286.

Thompson, A., Barley, M., Sullivan, S., et al. (2005) A pragmatic cluster randomised trial of the effect of a complex ward-based intervention on antipsychotic polypharmacy prescribing in adult psychiatric inpatient wards. UK Mental Health Research Network. National Scientific Conference, Manchester.

Thompson, C. (1994) The use of high-dose antipsychotic medication (consensus statement). *British Journal of Psychiatry*, **164**, 448–458.

Turner, J., Gardner, B., Staples, P. & Chapman, J. (2007) Medicines with respect: developing an integrated collaborative approach to medication management. *Mental Health Nursing*, **27**(6), 16–19.

Turner, J., Gardner, B., Staples, P. & Chapman, J. (2008) Medicines with respect: developing an integrative collaborative approach to medication management (2). *Mental Health Nursing*, **28**(7), 11–14.

Usher, K. & Arthur, D. (1998) Process consent: a model for enhancing informed consent in mental health nursing. *Journal of Advanced Nursing*, **27**, 692–697.

Usher, K., Lindsay, D. & Sellen, J. (2001) Mental health nurses' PRN psychotropic medication administration practices. *Journal of Psychiatric & Mental Health Nursing*, **8**(5), 383–390.

Vitiello, B., Ricciuti, A.J. & Behar, D. (1987) P.R.N. medications in child state hospital inpatients. *Journal of Clinical Psychiatry*, **48**(9), 351–354.

Walsh, S. (1996) Adapting cognitive analytic therapy to make sense of psychologically harmful work environments. *British Journal of Medical Psychology*, **69**, 3–20.

Waraich, P.S., Adams, C.E., Roque, M., Hamill, K.M. & Marti, J. (2002) Haloperidol dose for the acute phase of schizophrenia. In: *Cochrane Database of Systematic Reviews (3) Art No.: CD001951.*

Warner, J., Slade, R. & Barnes, T. (1995) Change in neuroleptic prescribing practice. *Psychiatric Bulletin*, **19**, 237–239.

Whittington, D. & McLaughlin, C. (2000) Finding time for patients: an exploration of nurses' time allocation in an acute psychiatric setting. *Journal of Psychiatric and Mental Health Nursing*, **7**, 259–268.

Wynaden, D., Chapman, R., McGowan, S., Holmes, C., Ash, P. & Boschman, A. (2002) Through the eye of the beholder: to seclude or not to seclude. *International Journal of Mental Health Nursing*, **11**, 260–268.

Yorston, G. & Pinney, A. (1997) Use of high dose antipsychotic medication. *Psychiatric Bulletin*, **21**, 566–569.

Index

Note: page numbers in *italics* refer to figures, those in **bold** refer to tables and boxes. Page numbers with suffix 'n' refer to footnotes.